help more of us to be great; to do both what's right and the right things for patients, and to make a real difference to every patient we come into contact with no matter how fleetingly.

**Audrey M Paterson**
*Director of Professional Policy,*
*The Society and College of Radiographers*
*Professor, Canterbury Christ Church University*

# Foreword

From my earliest days as a paramedic in Auckland, I knew the importance of strong, fair and open leadership and I witnessed firsthand the impact this had on individuals, teams and the organisation as a whole. I had some excellent role models in those early years, and this created a thirst for knowledge about different management styles and models of leadership.

I gained my knowledge primarily through reading and have over the years developed my own clear views on leadership, primary amongst those being the fundamentals of authenticity, resilience, compassion and the leader as servant. I see these reflected in various chapters of this excellent book, and was excited to read the 'head, heart and gut' section which resonated so strongly with my own experiences of leading people and projects.

I believe we are all in a state of continuing personal development, whether consciously or unconsciously, and the messages in Suzanne's book about the development of the individual and the organisation clearly sets out the impact of strong leadership on health outcomes. We have all seen the disastrous effects a lack of effective leadership can have on individuals and indeed whole systems over recent years.

I commend this book to colleagues across the health system who want to develop their thinking and understanding on some of the most up-to-date and healthcare relevant ideas on leadership today. The benefits for our people and our patients are too compelling to ignore.

**Peter Bradley CBE, MBA**
*CEO St John, New Zealand*

# Preface

This book is part of a journey—a personal journey of development and discovery, where through excellent teachers and challenging life and work lessons, I have, over time, developed a real passion for leadership. But not any leadership—leadership which is authentic and sincere, focussed on a way forward; leadership which is ethical and compassionate, which comes from a place of integrity, and which has within it a genuine desire for growth and positive change for all those involved, be that for ourselves, the colleagues we work with or the patients we serve. It is a leadership that is prepared to put personal ego aside to ensure the greater good of others and the service we work within. It is a leadership that wants to make a real difference and will do what it takes to ensure that the goal is reached within an ethical and compassionate framework.

To bring others along on that journey, this book introduces people with whom I have connected over the last few years, who have inspired me and shown me what this real, authentic and compassionate leadership is all about. The authors here have all shown real leadership in their own walks of professional life, are all passionate about what they do for others and are generous enough to share their learning to assist others in their ongoing leadership development.

The focus of the book is twofold: firstly, to assist personal leadership development, for personal satisfaction and growth, and secondly, to improve healthcare delivery to patients, through excellence in personal practice. I believe that it is through the passion, ability and drive of individuals (you and me) that we will change and challenge practices to ensure that patients get the best possible care in all healthcare contexts. It is not about spending more money or having more resources; it is about a genuine passion from within, a drive to give the best of ourselves driven by a sincere concern for those we serve through our careers. That is, I believe, how we will improve the quality of care and the quality of the work environment. It is then, I believe, as much about your intention, as your actions. I hope you are reading this book because you want to make even more of a difference, driven by respect and value of yourself and others: a compassionate desire to make things better.

## About This Book

This book is written to take you from where you are now to a new place on your leadership development journey. Whether you are already leading a large healthcare organisation, running your own practice, or are newly qualified (or not yet qualified), this book can assist you to take the next steps. We offer our thoughts, guided reflections, case studies and action points to enable you to fully engage with the ideas. Be prepared to challenge yourself and enjoy the process. (You might want to purchase a notebook to accompany your reading, as there is a real opportunity here to begin a leadership journal through the tools and activities outlined in the chapters to come.) Do come back and communicate with us about your experiences of using the tools and activities in the following chapters. Together, we can make a difference. We would love to hear how you apply what you read in your practice.

Let me introduce you to the authors and what they will be sharing:

Chapter 1.    Eileen Piggot-Irvine, myself and Paul Tosey begin by looking at what leadership is. While we look at the evolution of leadership over time and how thinking has moved, we focus on what we believe to be the way forward for leadership in health care. This chapter sets the scene, giving you the background you need to fully engage with the chapters to follow.

Chapter 2.    Daksha Malik, Dee Wilkinson and I then explore the issue of self-awareness and understanding in leadership, our belief being that self-awareness is the first and central step to leading yourself and consequently changing how you lead others.

Chapter 3.    Karen Moxom and Donna Blinston follow on the focus on self by exploring how we create a compelling vision and really understand what we want to achieve and where we want to go: setting a personal direction.

Chapter 4.    Lisa Booth and I share some ideas on communication excellence in preparation for you wanting to share your new understanding of self and your vision with others.

Chapter 5.    David Collier and Jennifer Haven then begin to explore beyond ourselves, as we look at taking this learning and applying it to how we lead others.

Chapter 6.    Sue Mellor looks specifically then at leadership of teams, a core skill in any healthcare context and one that is particularly relevant in today's health care of shifting professional boundaries and the increasing role of collaboration in multidisciplinary teams.

Chapter 7.    Maryann Hardy, Bev Snaith and I then pick up the issue of challenging professional boundaries, raising discussion around the changing culture of health care and the impact of these changes on current leadership required.

Chapter 8.  Melody Cheal and Joe Cheal further explore the challenges of leading change within an organisation, introducing concepts such as organisational fit, the political context of health care as a business, and working within policies and with a range of stakeholders.

Chapter 9.  Mark Klaassen introduces the concept of second-order leadership, which challenges us to think again about how we understand and lead change effectively by looking at it in a different way.

Chapter 10.  David Collier and Anna McNaughton take this new-found leadership confidence and sense of purpose and explore how you then inspire others to follow your lead.

Chapter 11.  Bev Snaith and Maryann Hardy then apply this directly to focusing change on driving and ensuring the quality of healthcare practice.

Chapter 12.  Denise Bancroft then shares some ideas for learning from experience. As we begin to push change forward, we have to be able to reflect deeply to evaluate whether or not the changes have been effective and to constantly learn from our own behaviours about the process as well as the outcome.

Chapter 13.  Joseph Quinn, Anna McNaughton and I then offer some practical skills in coaching which may be required at this stage to ensure all staff are engaged with your new vision and feel able to contribute effectively.

Chapter 14.  Joe Cheal and Melody Cheal take you to the next step of writing realistic and achievable goals to set out the direction upon which you have now agreed. This is an opportunity for you to explore what you will do as a result of reading and reflecting on leadership.

Chapter 15.  Gerri Power then offers you essential advice around resilience skills to keep you going when things get difficult and people oppose progress. Without the ability to carry on, and to keep going, many leaders stop driving forward before reaching their desired destination.

Chapter 16.  Grant Soosalu and I conclude with a short summary to bring together the main thoughts, to share an exciting new development and to encourage you to keep moving forward.

Just reviewing the contents again makes me excited, and I hope that sense of excitement and possibility comes across to you as you read this book.

The fact that you are reading this book already means that you want to do even more; you want to lead even more effectively; and you want to create a different future for you, for your team, your profession and hopefully your patients. You have already got ideas of how to improve things, and you already care enough to do something about it. That really excites me, and I hope you will take the contents of this book and add it to your own personal excellence to make your goals a reality. Together we can make changes one step at a time, constantly ensuring excellence at the point of delivery, always mindful of the patient as the focus—delivering care as we would want to be cared for.

Throughout the book we encourage you to stop and reflect on what you have read and to actively engage with the exercises and reflections we share with you. We want you to apply the ideas to your own area of practice and critique and evaluate what we have said, play with the materials and see how far you can take them. We want the book to stimulate discussion and enhance understanding of leadership excellence in practice. We want you to create the chapters not yet written, showing how practice continues to evolve and improve as you interact with and grow the materials further. So we would love for you to come back to us and let us know how you have used the book, what difference it has made and how you have developed the ideas further, as you keep coming back to the book to use it again in a new way.

It is our sincere hope that this book inspires you, excites you and supports you to be all the professional you can be. You are the leaders of today and of tomorrow, and you can create services to be proud of: care that is exceptional and truly touches and makes a difference to those who receive it. We hope this book will help you to do that in a real and practical way. Collectively we can create the change we want to see, and it is humbling and inspiring that you are reading this book to reflect on and improve your practice. Thank you for taking the time to read it, interact with it and apply it where you know it is appropriate to do so in your own field to complement what you already do really well. It is our desire that all patients will be cared for by people like you, people who care enough to see if they can even make just a small change to keep striving towards even greater levels of excellence: people who are willing to keep learning, keep developing and keep working hard to make good things happen. Thank you. We hope that through reading and interacting with this book, not only will you make positive change, you will also reflect on what you already do well so you can role model it to those following close behind you.

# About the Editor

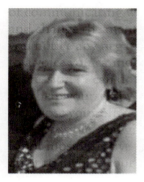

**Suzanne Henwood**, HDCR, PGCE, MSc, PhD, mANLP

Suzanne is a UK diagnostic radiographer by professional background and has worked in **higher** education (HE) almost continually since 1990 (with two short breaks working with a major **UK** health charity and running her own business). **At** the time of writing this book, she was an associate professor at Unitec in Auckland, in the Faculty **of** Social and Health Sciences, with a special interest in research and leadership, whilst also maintaining her coaching, consultancy and training work independently. Suzanne is a Neuro-Linguistic Programming (NLP) and multiple Brain Integration Techniques (mBIT) trainer and coach and works internationally in business and health care in the field of NLP, communication, leadership, transformational change, research and professional development. She is the author (and editor) of numerous books, book chapters and academic publications. She is the deputy editor of *Current Research in NLP* (published by ANLP), a founding and ongoing committee member of the International NLP Research Conference (hosted bi-annually by ANLP) and the associate editor (education) for the *Journal of Medical Radiation Sciences*. In 2013 Suzanne began working with mBraining International to promote and develop the new field of mBraining, establishing her company, mBraining4success, offering training, **coaching** and consultancy work with professionals to awaken, empower and **evolve** practice. Contact Suzanne at Suzanne@mBraining4success.com

# Contributors

**Denise Bancroft**, DTM, MPhil

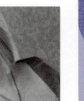

Denise has worked in the field of adult learning for over 20 years, specialising in leadership development. Although born in New Zealand, she worked in L&D in the UK for many years, consulting with leadership teams all over the UK. Denise has worked in leadership roles herself, and has always been involved in organisational development, both in the UK and NZ. She has managed or belonged to many project teams introducing strategic initiatives such as new performance review systems, online learning systems, and staff engagement surveys. While in the UK, Denise completed a master of philosophy at Henley Management College, majoring in adult experiential learning. Since returning to New Zealand, she has continued to work as an L&D consultant.

**Donna Blinston**

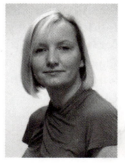

Donna is a certified trainer and master practitioner of NLP and time line comprehension, a life coach, a leadership and facilitation coach, and published author of two books *Psychobabble: A Straight Forward Plain English Guide to the Benefits of NLP* and *Make New Year's Resolutions and Keep Them Using NLP*. Donna is the host of *The NLP View* radio show, a unique, live, interactive, Internet talk-radio show that discusses the benefits of self-help through NLP. By professional background, Donna is a registered nurse, specialized in the field of gastroenterology and the liver. Donna developed within her nursing practice, gaining experience and qualification to her current role today as a nurse specialist in blood-borne viruses. As a certified trainer of NLP, she uses the tools and techniques of NLP to build a professional relationship with and enhance the lives of her patients to promote good health and well-being.

**Lisa Booth**

Dr Lisa Booth is a senior lecturer at the University of Cumbria, UK. Her research concerns patient care in radiography, and she has a special interest in the work of Eric Berne and his theory Transactional Analysis. Her career over the last 20 years includes clinical radiography as well as working in academia. She was awarded her PhD in 2002, and her thesis was titled *Communication Strategies in*

*Diagnostic Radiography: A Transactional Analysis Approach*. Since that time she has been an active member of the research committee for the Society of Radiography and chair of the North West Research Ethics Committee (NHS). She has supervised and examined a number of PhDs who focus on patient care in radiography, including breaking bad news in prenatal ultrasound and informed consent in prenatal ultrasound, and more recently has developed an interest in leadership.

**Joe Cheal**, MSc, BA (Hons), NLP Master Trainer

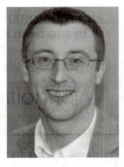

Joe holds an MSc in organisational development and neurolinguistic technologies and a joint BA(Hons)degree in philosophy and psychology. He is an NLP master trainer, an Emotional Intelligence (EI) practitioner and an Institute of Leadership and Management (ILM) accredited trainer. He is a partner in the GWiz Learning Partnership, and as a trainer, coach and consultant he has inspired others to achieve outstanding results. Since 1993, he has worked with a broad range of organisational cultures, helping thousands of people revolutionise the way they work with others. With a passion and a penchant for the nature of paradox, Joe has published a book entitled *Solving Impossible Problems: Working through Tensions and Paradox in Business*. His MSc dissertation was an exploration into 'social paradox', and his findings were published in the first *NLP Research Journal* in 2009. He is also the creator and editor of the ANLP journal *Acuity*.

**Melody Cheal**, MS, BA, NLP Master Trainer

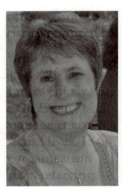

Melody has a BA degree in psychology, a master's degree in applied positive psychology, a diploma in psychotherapy and is a certified NLP master trainer. She is a member of the external verification panel for the ANLP accreditation programme. She is also a qualified Myers Briggs practitioner and EI practitioner and has had 5 years Transactional Analysis training, meaning she is able to help organisations access the hidden potential in their staff. She is also in demand for her work in transforming average or even troubled teams into high performers. As a partner in the GWiz Learning Partnership, Melody runs courses in both the private and the public sectors, focusing on interpersonal skills and self-awareness. Over the last 20 years she has worked with international committees, directors, senior managers, teams and front-line staff in groups and one-to-one as a coach. She is also an ILM-accredited trainer.

**David Collier**, MA (Hons), Dip Tchg, Dip Cns

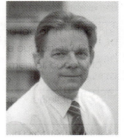

David was appointed chief executive of the Australian Institute of Radiography (AIR) in June 2008. He began his working life in New Zealand with varied roles in social work, teaching and as an assistant lecturer at Auckland University. After getting married, he took on a position as a press secretary for the NZ government before starting a career in consulting in 1992. In 1997 he relocated to Australia and took up a role as the principal consultant for the Compliance Management Group Pty Ltd (Australia) in 1998, working predominantly in the healthcare sector in knowledge, compliance management and delivery, leadership, and governance. In 2003 he joined the Royal Australian and New Zealand College of Psychiatrists as the manager of training, assessment and examinations, and in 2004 he became the CEO/registrar of the Psychologists Registration Board of Victoria, working in four areas of activity: registration, complaints investigation, development and education, and administration.

**Maryann Hardy**, PhD, MSc, BSc (Hons), DCR(R)

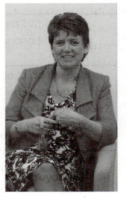

Maryann qualified as a diagnostic radiographer in 1989 and worked as a clinical radiographer for 9 years before entering academia as a lecturer in 1998. In 2002 she became the first radiographer to be awarded a Department of Health doctoral research fellowship for a study considering the epidemiology of children's injuries. She was promoted to chair of radiography and imaging practice research at the University of Bradford in 2009 and is a widely published author and international speaker in her field. Her research focuses specifically on service improvement through practice innovation.

**Jennifer Haven**

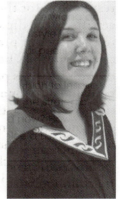

Jennifer graduated with a BSc (Hons) in diagnostic radiography from the University of Leeds in 2006. She took her first professional role at Birmingham Children's Hospital and completed a post-graduate certificate in nuclear medicine from the University of West England. Following 2 years of practice in the UK National Health Service, Jennifer made the move to New Zealand with a sense of excitement and anticipation. In New Zealand, Jennifer has enjoyed radiography roles in both the public and private sector for adult and paediatric patients. A passion for education then led her to join the Unitec Institute of Technology team as a clinical tutor, a lecturer and now the programme leader for the Bachelor of Health Science (Medical Imaging) programme. During this time, Jennifer has continued her own education at Unitec, and she was recently awarded a first class honours degree for the master of health science (medical radiation technology).

## Mark Klaassen

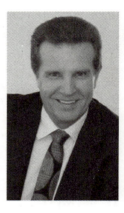

Director of communications plus international NLP (CPI), Mark is a certified NLP master trainer (INLPTA), professional facilitator and business consultant to some of New Zealand's largest companies, including Air New Zealand, ASB Bank, Fletchers, Vodafone and Fonterra. His background in human development, change, finance, and business growth has given him a dynamic understanding of the 'X factors' needed for business and personal success. Also training NLP certifications for professional and personal development, Mark is qualified in several areas of human development and personal change; he utilises and teaches skills in NLP, spiral dynamics, the enneagram, business leadership, executive development and performance coaching.

## Daksha Malik

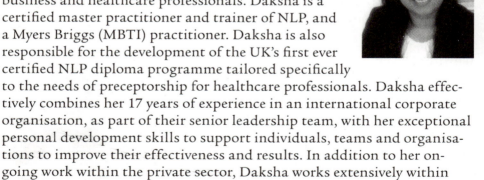

Daksha is the owner of Unique Minds Ltd. and is a personal development coach and trainer specialising in the provision of NLP coaching and training to business and healthcare professionals. Daksha is a certified master practitioner and trainer of NLP, and a Myers Briggs (MBTI) practitioner. Daksha is also responsible for the development of the UK's first ever certified NLP diploma programme tailored specifically to the needs of preceptorship for healthcare professionals. Daksha effectively combines her 17 years of experience in an international corporate organisation, as part of their senior leadership team, with her exceptional personal development skills to support individuals, teams and organisations to improve their effectiveness and results. In addition to her ongoing work within the private sector, Daksha works extensively within the public/healthcare sector developing and delivering a wide range of interventions, including leadership development at all levels, transitional change, communications, preceptorship and dementia care, to name but a few.

**Anna McNaughton**, GradCertCareerDev, GDHE, PGDipSocS

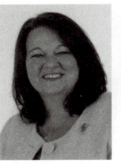

Anna is an experienced facilitator, manager and coach with 20 years of experience developing people of all ages and backgrounds. She has incredible energy and wealth of knowledge, having worked in a wide range of organisations on a range of projects. Whilst Anna's career started in health, she has also worked as a project manager, management consultant and corporate trainer. She works for Grafton Consulting Limited as a senior consultant and leads their Grafton Assist Team, which is an HR consultancy service. Previously she was the national learning and development manager for a large health-care organization. Anna is senior practitioner/manager with experience in health services in Australia and New Zealand. She provides staff and manager development to many organisations in New Zealand and is experienced in providing corporate training from boardroom to factory floor. She has experience in change processes through individual coaching, career development and supporting organisational processes. Anna is a master NLP practitioner and accredited in MBTI and LSI/GSI.

**Sue Mellor**

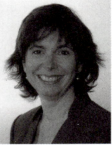

Sue originally specialized in theatre nursing, where she became fascinated with the synergy of effective team working and the ever-changing team dynamics. In 2001 she led the team coaching training for the National Clinical Governance Support Team, coaching executive leaders and teams through change, conflict and service redesign while also supporting the Department of Health. She is now a director for SMM Coaching & Consultancy Ltd, presenting for the NHS Institute and speaks at national conferences on teams and human factors. She is an accredited mediator, human factors trainer and coach supervisor. She is an NLP practitioner and has a master's degree from Oxford Brookes University in research in coaching and mentoring in practice, focusing on coaching teams through merger. Sue is passionate about cultural transformation through creative leadership to improve the patient experience.

**Karen Moxom**, BSc (Hons), PTLLS, Certified Trainer of NLP

Karen is the managing director of the Association for NLP, an independent award-winning social enterprise specialising in membership services for NLP professionals. She is motivated to do the best she can to help NLP become more credible so that it will be embraced by healthcare professionals, the education system and businesses, so more people will be empowered to reach their full potential. As well as running ANLP, Karen is the author of *The NLP Professional*; is the editor of *Rapport*, the magazine for NLP professionals; and is the publisher of *Acuity* and the NLP Research Journal, *Current Research in NLP*. Karen is an assistant district commissioner with the Scout Association and she is part of the 'developing special provision locally parent reference group' for Hertfordshire County Council. She was awarded Hertfordshire Woman of the Year in the 2009 Hertfordshire Business Awards.

### Eileen Piggot-Irvine

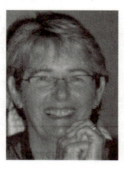

Eileen is a professor of leadership at Royal Roads University, Canada, and an adjunct professor at Griffith University, Brisbane, and at Unitec, Auckland. She was formerly director of the New Zealand Action Research and Review Centre (NZARRC), director of the New Zealand Principal and Leadership Centre (NZPLC) and senior lecturer at Massey University. Prior to 1998 she was the head of the Education Management Centre at Unitec, Auckland, and head of professional development at Northland Polytechnic. Her current research, evaluations and publications are in the fields of appraisal/performance evaluation, leadership development, organizational learning, action research, success case methodology, and management review. She has published four books, multiple book chapters, and approximately 50 journal articles and presented too many keynotes, etc., to count. She is currently the editor for an international action research monograph series. In the last 6 years she has directed 11 evaluation contracts (several at a national level), and all have had a strongly collaborative, action research-influenced approach.

### Gerri Power

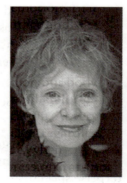

Gerri Power, a certified master coach and mentor based in Auckland, New Zealand, provides an integrative, whole-brain approach to developing resilient leadership to a diverse mix of corporate, health, education and not-for-profit organisations. An accredited HBDI® practitioner and mBIT coach, Gerri has a background in organisational development and more than 20 years consulting experience. Her areas of expertise include leader and team development with a focus on workplace resilience and well-being, both from the individual and organisational perspectives. An area of special interest to Gerri is the emerging field of research-based practices in writing for insight, creativity and well-being in the context of leadership challenges. She has trained extensively in this approach and her work is enriched through these studies and as a hospice life story facilitator. Inspired by the resilience of the human spirit, a key focus for Gerri is coaching individuals and teams in finding deeper meaning and purpose in their professional and personal lives during times of change and transition.

**Joseph Quinn**, certified trainer of NLP and hypnosis, Dip performance coaching

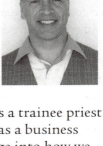

Joseph is the owner of a communication skills company called Influencing Now that creates skilled, resourceful and proactive influencers from managers, supervisors and leaders who enable growth and development in others. His company also specialises in offering international certifications in Neuro-Linguistic Programming (NLP). Throughout his career as a trainee priest in Ireland, 10 years as a police officer in the UK and now as a business owner, he has gained significant experience and knowledge into how we, as individuals, can expand our thinking and behaviours. Joseph believes that people *want* and *can* achieve greater results with authentic influence, and he thrives on working with them to do just that. Consulting for government, corporate and NGO organisations, as well as coaching individuals, has afforded Joseph the opportunity of seeing change occur where it was needed. He believes that we each have greater abilities than we credit ourselves with and that authentic change happens when we get out there and use our skills.

**Bev Snaith**, PhD, MSc, FCR

Bev Snaith was appointed as one of the first allied health consultant roles in the UK in 2003 and still retains a full-time clinical radiographer role. She is responsible for the leadership of imaging services and radiographers across a multicentre NHS Trust and maintains honorary academic roles in a number of universities. She has maintained a strong presence within the professional body (Society and College of Radiographers), and was awarded an honorary fellowship in 2010. She is the author of a number of peer-reviewed papers and two textbooks and is an editorial board member for the

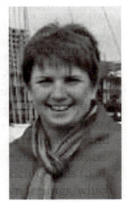

journal *Radiography*. The main focus of her work is on role development and service innovation and has recently been awarded a PhD by Published Work.

**Grant Soosalu**, MAppSc, BSc (Hons), Grad Dip Psych, NLP master practitioner, certified master behavioural modeller

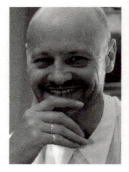

Grant Soosalu is a co-developer of the newly emerging field of mBIT (multiple Brain Integration Techniques). mBIT is being hailed as a groundbreaking synthesis of the latest research in neurology and cognitive science, and a true advancement of the field of NLP. Grant is an experienced trainer, leadership consultant and executive coach with extensive backgrounds in organisational change, training and leadership development. He has advanced degrees and certifications in applied physics, psychology, positive psychology, computer engineering and system development. He is a qualified Total Quality Management (TQM) trainer and has achieved master practitioner certification in the behavioural sciences of NLP and advanced behavioural modelling. More recently, Grant was awarded a graduate coaching diploma in the newly emerging field of authentic happiness coaching.

**Paul Tosey**, BSc, MSc, PhD

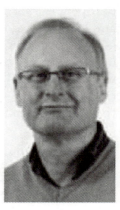

Paul is a senior lecturer at the University of Surrey Business School. His research concerns organisational learning and transformative learning, and he has a special interest in the work of Gregory Bateson, who was a seminal influence on the developers of NLP. His career experience over 30 years includes consultancy, coaching and line management. He was awarded a national teaching fellowship by the Higher Education Academy in 2007. Paul is an active member of the University Forum for Human Resource Development (HRD) and currently chairs its Programme and Qualification Activities Committee. He has encouraged and supported a research-minded approach in the field of NLP and convened the first International NLP Research Conference in 2008. Most recently he has been exploring clean language, an innovative coaching practice that is based on metaphor, both as a researcher and as a trained facilitator.

### Dee Wilkinson

Dee is one of the most respected and sought-after coaches both within and outside the NHS with a wealth of NHS experience. She has gained this reputation based on her professionalism, credibility, integrity and ability to connect with her clients. Since completing her training in 2004, she has over 1000 hours of coaching experience. Dee now specialises in General Practitioner (GP) coaching. Within the NHS she also coaches consultants, executive directors, senior managers and team leaders. Using a systems perspective, linked with a genuine passion and coaching presence, she gets results 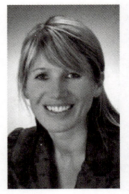 very quickly. As well as a coach, Dee is a qualified supervisor, trainer and facilitator with 20 years of NHS experience in leading innovative teams, transforming working methods, building personal skills and inspiring people. Dee's focus is on aligning the vision and energy of individuals with the needs of the organisation—transforming both. Dee now runs her own business, South West Coaching Ltd.

# 1 Introduction to Leadership

Eileen Piggot-Irvine, Suzanne Henwood and Paul Tosey

## Introduction: The Need for a New Style of Leadership

As we launch into what we hope will become a core and favourite book of yours, one that is well thumbed and referred to over and over in the coming years, we focus in this introductory chapter on what leadership is to us so that we can begin on the same page.

A number of authors suggest that the need for leadership (and leadership development) in health care is now a priority. We would go further to suggest that not only good leadership, but also a new paradigm of leadership is essential to ensure the future of health care at a quality we are all proud of. We are supported by other authors: The UK Chartered Institute for Personnel and Development (2012) reported to members that 'a new type of leadership is needed in modern organisations in order to build positive workplace cultures that get the best out of people and support innovation, empowerment and ethical behaviour'. The Kings Fund (2012), in a leadership review in health care in the UK, also proposed that a new style of leadership is required.

Contemporary thinking about leadership demonstrates an emphasis on leadership as a collaborative and relational activity that generates high openness and trust, with a shared responsibility, and no longer focuses on one person as 'leader'. It is, if you like, all to do with purposeful influence, within a specific context, through relationship, driven by a desire for service improvement, not personal gain. It is based on integrity, trust, honesty and a deep connection to relationship with others in order (in health care) to enhance service delivery and patient care through deep and authentic engagement. This latest thinking encompasses an assumption that the roles of global healthcare practitioners are changing, and that each person needs to 'step up' and play their part in ensuring quality and making change happen. Leadership in practice is now everyone's responsibility and needs to be at all levels, working across all boundaries (Welbourne et al. 2012). It is no longer appropriate to sit back and assume someone else will take the lead.

Within an increasingly complex and constantly evolving healthcare environment, there has never been a more critical time to look at leadership effectiveness. If this is what excites you, drives you, concerns you, attracts you, or even just intrigues you, and especially if this stance underpins your work, then read on.

## What Is Leadership?

If you have ever googled *leadership* as a topic, you know that you will get a list of hits in the millions. It is an enormous topic that has multiple interpretations and definitions, with added complexity in health care around two complementary issues: leadership and clinical leadership. As Howieson and Thiagarajah (2011, 7) report, there is 'widespread fascination with leadership maybe because it is such a mysterious process, as well as one that touches everyone's life'. They also suggest that it is a black box because it has so many elements that are unexplainable. However, we aim to offer some key interpretations within a contemporary healthcare context.

We begin by stating that leadership is viewed very differently today compared with the past. Previously, leadership was often associated with individual authority figures who wielded power based on their position in a hierarchy, or with 'heroes' who led through their personal impact. Leadership has also been linked to traits, charisma, roles, personality, behaviours, ethics and power—the list is almost endless.

Today, there is much more emphasis on relationships, influence, adaptability and complexity. As Davidson (2010, 108) says,

> The leadership structures of the twentieth century were based on hierarchical and linear models.... Simply stated, these mechanistic models of leadership failed to capture or account for the highly complex, interrelated, relationship-driven organisations that have become the reality of the twenty-first century.

In health care, this moves us away from a traditional model of hierarchy and individual or medical dominance towards one of shared, collaborative or distributed leadership, respecting and valuing the role that each and every team member and every health discipline plays in delivering excellent health care. Moreover, leadership is less now about the capabilities of one person, but about a process, heavily contextualised, with shared control to achieve the desired outcomes. Leadership is now the responsibility of all staff, whether or not they occupy a formal leadership role.

# Distinguishing Management and Leadership

Another important issue to consider is the differences and similarities between *management* and *leadership*. Sometimes the terms are used interchangeably. Traditionally, though, a distinction has often been made between the tasks of management, which include organising, controlling and planning, and those of leadership, which describes the long-term, big-picture, strategic work. There is a growing tendency, however, to expect managers to provide leadership (as well as for many leaders to perform some management functions). This means that elements of leadership are implicit in both these roles, regardless of whether they are formally classified as management or leadership roles within the organisational structure.

We also believe that *both* leadership and management are important. You may have worked with a leader who was exceptionally visionary but had poor management skills. Such lack of organisation can drive staff to distraction. Equally frustrating is someone who micromanages, organizes and controls to excess, without inspiring and empowering staff to thrive and effect change. We believe a balance or close relationship between these two functions is required, with healthy respect for both.

As health care professionals, we believe that *all* practitioners lead—within certain spheres of influence—as part of their normal practice. In addition, new roles such as advanced and consultant therapists are challenged with creating new leadership roles in clinical care, which are further stretching the definitions of clinical leadership in practice across the health professions.

In order to further develop this new conception of leadership we consider three major themes in more detail. These are:

1. The importance of influence

2. Relational and authentic leadership

3. Leadership as pragmatic and contextual

## The Importance of Influence

*Influence* is a term often associated with leadership (Kelloway and Barling 2010; Northouse 2004; Welbourne et al. 2012; Yukl 2006). For example, Yukl (2002) considers that leaders 'influence' interpretation of events, choice of outcomes, organisation of work, motivation and abilities of individuals. According to Cummings et al. (2008, p. 240), 'The following elements are central to the definition of leadership: leadership (a) is a process; (b) entails influence; (c) occurs within a group setting or context; and (d) involves achieving goals that reflect a common vision'.

Of course there is a potentially darker side to influence, such as influence without integrity, or influence for personal gain. Daft and Pirola-Merlo (2009, p. 115) warn that inappropriate use of charisma to 'influence', for example, can 'be used for self-serving purposes, which leads to deception, manipulation and exploitation of others...it is potentially dangerous'. In this book we emphasise the need for ethical influence that is appropriate in process and intent, driven by a patient-centred focus and a desire to enhance the quality of service delivery.

### REFLECTION

- What do the words *authority* and *influence* mean to you in a leadership context?

- Thinking of specific leaders and contexts, can you identify what constitutes positive and negative authority and influence?

- What role do you believe authority and influence have for leadership in today's healthcare context?

## Relational Leadership

Much contemporary research resonates with the idea that leadership is largely *a social and relational process*. For example, Cummings et al. (2008, p. 247) looked at factors associated with leadership effectiveness in a clinical setting. Their findings suggest that 'characteristics such as transformational, high relationship styles and previous leadership experience are identified as contributing to leadership qualities'.

Daniel Goleman (2000, 2006) has written several books over recent years highlighting the need for leaders to have 'emotional intelligence' and more recently 'social intelligence'. These views have proved to be very influential, although it is important to note that the concept of `emotional intelligence' and the benefits being claimed for it by some proponents are being questioned by some researchers (e.g., Clarke 2006), especially the idea that it represents some kind of panacea. We support a pragmatic view, where emotional intelligence is *one* of the components that it is useful to explore when critically reflecting on leadership.

Goleman (2006) argues (with input from Johnson and Indvik [1999]) that effective leaders require competences across four core areas:

- *Self-awareness* (self-assessment, self-confidence): The ability to recognise our own emotions, know the causes of these emotions and recognise the difference between feelings and actions
- *Self-management* (self-control, transparency, adaptability, achievement, initiative, optimism): The ability to tolerate frustration, manage anger and suspend judgement
- *Relationship management* (inspiration, influence, teamwork, collaboration, developing others, conflict management, change catalyst): Includes the capacity to find common ground and build rapport
- *Social awareness* (empathy, organisational awareness, service): The capacity to understand the emotional makeup of others and treat people accordingly

Goleman's (2006) work considerably shifted thinking about leadership effectiveness towards 'knowing ourselves and our responses to others' as leaders. Interestingly, Johnson and Indvik (1999) report that 80% of success of leaders can be attributed to emotional intelligence, with the essential element being a sense of self-awareness. Self-awareness, however, does not sit in isolation and, in turn, creates capacity to exercise self-control when problems arise. Goleman (2000, p. 85) outlines what is required to develop emotional intelligence:

- A desire to change
- Self-reflection
- Listening to one's internal script
- Developing emotional control
- Practising empathy and listening skills
- Validating the emotions of others

## REFLECTION

- How would you score yourself (out of 10) against the four areas of emotional intelligence? Compare those scores with how your colleagues would score you.
- What areas could you develop further to increase your emotional intelligence over time? How might you go about that development?

## Values-Based Leadership

A related theme of 'values-based leadership' is currently also strongly supported as being associated with organisational effectiveness (Fein, Vasiliu, and Tziner 2011; Meglino and Ravlin 1998; Schaubroeck, Lam, and Cha 2007). Values-based leadership is echoed in an important strand of work on authentic leadership (Avolio and Gardner 2005). Levy and Bentley's (2007) ideas on this theme are that authentic leadership involves leaders in:

- Making decisions based on core values
- Saying exactly what they mean
- Analysing relevant data before deciding
- Making difficult decisions based on high standards of ethical conduct
- Admitting mistakes when they are made
- Seeking feedback to improve interactions with others
- Accurately describing how others view their capabilities
- Soliciting views that challenge deeply held positions

Levy and Bentley (2007) believe that authentic leaders are passionate about their purpose, practice and values. They are not only self-disciplined; they also combine leading with their hearts and heads. For such leaders, meaningful relationships are important, and we would argue that this style of leadership is only possible alongside a high degree of self-awareness (an issue we explore further in Chapter 2) and an openness to feedback that enables continuous improvement over time, which takes courage and determination.

## Leadership as Pragmatic and Contextual

The shift in leadership theory in the twenty-first century is towards more relational styles of leadership which have fluidity and adaptability for a rapidly changing environment, where it is important 'to thrive amongst the unknown' (Davidson 2010, p. 109).

Further evolution is occurring to more-complex adaptive, systemic, quantum, blended or, as we like to think, more *pragmatic leadership*, which recognises the complex and organic nature of leadership within specific contexts and takes the best practice of all that has gone before and utilises what works for the practice context being considered. It requires both the knowledge of the science of leadership as well as expertise in the practice of the art of leadership.

What is also clear is that leadership can work at all levels (individual, team, organisational, local, national, global, within and across professional boundaries) and that, at any one time, we may be acting across many of those categories simultaneously. An effective leader will keep an overview of the whole system and the impacts of any changes introduced. (Systems thinking is considered further in Chapter 9.)

Effective leaders are flexible and adaptable, able to stand back and visualise systemic change and modify their behaviours to ensure continuous movement towards their desired vision. They also have the ability to predict future changes and prepare systems to meet future needs, along with the resilience to keep going regardless of obstacles along the way.

Goleman's (2000) work also suggests that effective leaders are able to employ a range of styles—an appropriate style at the right time in the right measure. This complements nicely our perspective of the need for *pragmatic leadership*, that is, using what works and having the capacity to flexibly move between styles to meet needs as they arise, in each context, whilst striving forward to meet desired outcomes.

## Summary: So What Is Leadership?

In summary, leadership as a notion is thought to be too complex and controversial to define in simple terms. Thinking about leadership has a long history involving many different and conflicting points of view.

For the purposes of this book, and in the changing, complex context of health care in the twenty-first century, leadership is something that all healthcare professionals are likely to need to develop. We believe that *influence* with a purposeful intent to generate positive change plays a central role in leadership; that it is a highly social and *relational* process that requires engagement, integrity and authenticity; and finally that it is heavily contextualised and pragmatic in order to suit the identified purposes and desired outcomes.

Having discussed our conception of leadership, the remaining sections of this chapter put these ideas into practice in order to help you in your journey towards becoming an even more confident and skilled leader. We have written this book to offer you some practical development and reflection opportunities around what we believe to be some of the core issues in leadership. Our aim is to share the experience of some of the current leaders in the field and the current thinking on leadership to further enhance healthcare service delivery and expert practice.

First we consider the question of 'What makes for effective leadership?' Then we explore the topic of productive reasoning as an antidote to the defensiveness that can inhibit authentic leadership. Finally we enable you to identify your preferred leadership style or styles before moving into the topics outlined in the proceeding chapters.

# What Is Effective Leadership?

Kouzes and Posner (2002) have repeatedly surveyed employees to determine what is expected of immediate leaders; consistently, the top four characteristics are honesty, forward looking, competence and inspiring. Williams (2004) found that to be effective, leaders in health care must be able to:

- Create strategy
- Have a vision for change
- Design new ways of working to respond to these changes
- Develop others
- Maintain morale while maximizing performance
- Work both within teams and across boundaries
- Focus on customers, both internal and external, and build relationships with them

Many of these features of effectiveness emphasise leadership as both strategic and relational. While characteristics alone do not define leadership excellence, they are one component worth considering when exploring leadership effectiveness.

## REFLECTION

- What does effective leadership in health care look like to you?

## ACTIVITY

### Significant Features of Effective Leadership

Do a Google search on leadership characteristics and consider those that are most important to *you*. Do this on a rough piece of paper or sticky notes so that you can then prioritise these into a list of the 'top ten'. List your top ten in Table 1.1. Now score each item from 1 (low) to 5 (high) for how effective you currently perceive your leadership to be (in whatever context you lead).

Reflecting on your list, record which two are areas you would most like to improve and state how you can begin to develop those characteristics further in Table 1.2. What benefit would there be in pursuing that development?

Our guess is that it is very likely you will have listed characteristics associated with openness and honesty in your top ten list. These characteristics have invariably been listed when we have asked others to brainstorm the components of effectiveness. We think that it's important to declare our own view on openness by stating that it is associated with deeply complex

**Table 1.1:** My Top-Ten Characteristics of Effective Leadership

|  | Characteristic | Effectiveness ranking (1 = low; 5 = high) |
|---|---|---|
|  |  |  |
| 1 |  |  |
| 2 |  |  |
| 3 |  |  |
| 4 |  |  |
| 5 |  |  |
| 6 |  |  |
| 7 |  |  |
| 8 |  |  |
| 9 |  |  |
| 10 |  |  |

**Table 1.2:** Characteristics that Could Be Even Further Improved

|  | Development plan with timescale | Perceived benefits |
|---|---|---|
| Improvement area one: |  |  |
| Improvement area two: |  |  |

interactions linked to lowering control and 'power over others' as leaders. Therefore, we consider that *trust is a hard-earned outcome of openness* based on what is sometimes described as *productive reasoning* in leadership. The following section focuses on this element.

# Productive Reasoning

Underpinning much of the thinking about values-based, authentic leadership—and reinforcing the theme of emotional intelligence—is an emphasis on creating openness and trust between leaders and their staff. As we implied in the previous section, this does not happen by accident. It results from extremely complex interactions, at a one-to-one level, that are based on non-defensive (often called 'productive') values and strategies. It does not result from an emphasis on needing to be nice or liked! This is echoed by Chris Argyris, perhaps one of the most renowned experts in the psychology of effective work relationships. He says:

> The ability to get along with others is always an asset, right? Wrong. By adeptly avoiding conflict with co-workers, some executives eventually wreak organisational havoc. (Argyris 1986, p. 74)

Wreaking havoc by avoiding conflict is not confined to executives at the most senior level in organisations. Such avoidance exists at all levels of leadership and management, and sometimes it can be an indication of low self-esteem in a leader.

## REFLECTION

- Have you experienced defensive or avoidance behaviours in healthcare leadership? If yes, how has that behaviour affected your trust in the leadership?

- Describe the specific avoidance behaviours have you experienced (e.g., failing to come to the point about a concern, etc.).

- Which of these defensive avoidance behaviours do you recognise that you engage in when in a difficult or conflict situation?

Defensive behaviours go beyond just avoidance. They are also associated with control and abuse of power. It is sometimes useful to think of control and avoidance as two sides of the same defensive coin.

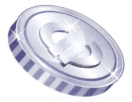

In fact, many avoidance behaviours can be interpreted as extremely manipulative control, even when the perpetrator is often unaware of that control element. An example might demonstrate this. If leaders avoid coming to the point about a concern (the example provided in the last reflection), they may be withholding information or, to put it another way, they could be failing to reveal important information that might help resolve the concern. Many would consider that leaders in this situation could superficially look like they are avoiding, but in fact they are also likely to be controlling what information to reveal. Keep in mind, therefore, that avoidance and control are the two key elements of defensiveness.

Interestingly, Argyris (1990), after observing thousands of people, has shown that such defensiveness is 'normal' behaviour in society, so it really is something we all need to learn how to manage. Argyris defines defensiveness as the tendency to protect ourselves and others from potential threat. He considers that we behave defensively by covering up or bypassing threat, being indirect with people, giving mixed messages, or withholding information. Defensiveness, he says, is an anti-learning process which can lead to misunderstandings, distortions, and ultimately ineffective teams and organisations. In our experience, the more-controlling elements of defensiveness are also strongly linked to abuse of power and align with perceptions of bullying.

What is most concerning is that defensiveness is often automatic behaviour that is usually below our level of consciousness, and it has its roots in our early childhood experiences. At this young stage of our lives—when we are instilled with the virtues of caring, helping, supporting and respecting others—such virtues, though laudable if used in moderation, can lead to avoidance of confronting issues if used to an extreme. An example should demonstrate this. If leaders are excessively caring or overly concerned about hurting the feelings of staff, this may prevent them from being clear about underperformance issues. Such 'avoiding' behaviour leads to ineffective leadership and an underperforming department and, eventually, an underperforming organisation. Another virtue that we are often conditioned with from childhood is that of sticking to our principles. Again, this is fine in moderation but destructive if overdone. Leaders who excessively stick to their principles may be inflexible in discussions, and this may come across to staff as 'controlling' behaviour that results in the power play and, ultimately, the bullying that we have already mentioned. Such behaviour also leads to ineffective teams and organisations. Avoidance and control are therefore the two major strategies of defensiveness, and increasing our self-awareness in relation to these strategies can be the first step to choosing to behave differently.

In order to overcome defensiveness, we must first look at the way that we *personally* engage in control and/or avoidance behaviours rather than blaming others. The next activity is designed to assist you to reveal your defensiveness in a conversation with a staff member.

## REFLECTION

- Think about a difficult conversation you have had with a staff member: What avoiding or controlling strategies did you use to get the outcome you desired?

- In hindsight, what could you have done differently that might ensure you did not slip into defensiveness?

Overcoming defensiveness can involve months, maybe years, of training (Piggot-Irvine 2012). The reason for this is that taking a different approach requires rethinking and altering our underlying value systems, and this involves changing many automatic, conditioned responses. Such values and responses can rarely be changed in a couple of hours! The role of appropriate high-quality leadership coaching can be invaluable to help development in this area, and we would argue that such development is unlikely to occur without such expert support. Overcoming defensiveness requires the adoption of values and strategies of productive reasoning, as summarised in Table 1.3.

We could also add two other features of productive reasoning which overlap with descriptions of the elements of good interpersonal

**Table 1.3:** Productive Reasoning

| Guiding values | Key strategies |
|---|---|
| Increase valid information for all (Advocacy) | When discussing issues with others:<br>• Share control by exposing, rather than withholding, key information; state your position clearly |
| | • Disclose your views and the evidence (data) that led to those views |
| | • Invite challenge, evaluation, and public testing of those views and be prepared to change them |
| Enhance freedom of informed choice (Enquiry) | • Treat views and reactions of yourself and others as hypotheses to be tested (rather than predetermined outcomes) |
| | • Check to see how views have been understood and what views others hold; encourage and non-defensively receive others' views and disagreements without pre-judgement; check perceptions in ways that reveal implicit and explicit assumptions |
| Gain internal commitment to choice and to monitoring (Bilateralism) | • Seek bilateral solutions and take joint responsibility for planning, implementing, and monitoring of achievement of goals |
| | • Manage difficult emotional issues as a joint responsibility |

*Source:* Piggot-Irvine (2001), adapted from Cardno (1994, p. 159).

relationships generally. These are the features of leaders (a) helping staff to feel appreciated and valued and (b) adopting listening and reporting skills based on confidentiality.

Productive reasoning involves a balancing act between the two predominant features of 'advocacy' and 'enquiry'. The overuse or underuse of either of these features can result in either controlling or avoidance strategies, that is, defensive strategies. Balanced advocacy and enquiry should create a genuine two-way dialogue, or informed debate, between leaders and staff which results in a mutual understanding and agreement about issues, even if the agreement is to disagree. Once this informed dialogue and authentic collaboration (Piggot-Irvine 2012) has occurred, then solutions to any issues can be mutually agreed upon, and improvements can be planned for, implemented and monitored in ways which enable individuals to be responsible for their own decisions. The critical elements of productive reasoning, according to Dick and Dalmau (1999, p. 47), include being 'more consensual, more open to change'.

Most leaders espouse, or say, that they are productive, but as we have suggested earlier, few employ these skills in problem situations where contention and threat are heightened. It is important to note that just changing the words that you use in developing productive skills will not be enough. Becoming candid and open while holding defensive values is a recipe for distrust and disaster. In order to live the values of productive reasoning, you need to change your underlying values! We believe it is the leader's role to set the culture and intention of the desired way of working by role modelling productive reasoning in practice. Again, we recommend appropriate leadership coaching as a mechanism for exploring and changing values in a safe environment. It is not something that will change without conscious effort.

## What Is Your Leadership Style?

Ideas about leadership *style* represent an important strand in thinking about leadership. There is a move away from the belief that there is one best way to lead, towards one in which leadership behaviours are dependent or contingent on the situation. Hence one of the best-known models of leadership style is 'situational leadership' (Hersey and Blanchard 1977). Recent health literature also stresses the need for the contextualisation of leadership (Kings Fund 2011) and the need to take into account all of the variables which impact on leadership effectiveness. The idea of style also shifts the emphasis from the personal traits of leaders towards their behavioural flexibility, the capacity to adapt style according to the context. This has a good fit with our emphasis on the pragmatic, contextual nature of leadership, along with the move away from hierarchical, heroic models, demonstrating a significant paradigm shift in leadership thinking.

Because of this move, we have decided to avoid including any inventory or checklist for analysing leadership style. Many such style inventories have been developed. If you have a strong need to use such an inventory, we would recommend the one developed by Bolton and Bolton (1984), which focuses on 'social style' within the concept of leadership. Though not using the terms, this inventory touches on some of the relational, values-based, and productive emphasis in leadership that we have previously noted by looking for 'a pervasive and enduring pattern of [your] interpersonal behaviours' (Bolton and Bolton 1984, p. 3), along with some suggestions about how to 'flex' a predominant style to be more adaptable to others with different styles (when known). This is in keeping with our earlier discussion of pragmatic and contextual leadership.

# How Can You Get the Most from This Book?

You have already started to experience how leadership can be developed and enhanced. You have also begun to reflect on your own strengths and to consider leadership within your own work context. We concur with many researchers such as Cummings et al. (2008) and Kouzes and Posner (2002), who believe that leadership can be learnt, a view that is shared by Goleman, Boyatzis, and McKee (2002, p. 101):

> Great leaders, the research shows, are made as they gradually acquire in the course of their lives and careers the competencies that make them so effective. The competencies can be learned by any leader, at any point.

Our experience as leaders, academics and as coaches abounds with examples of novice leaders incrementally growing, with the right support, in effectiveness as leaders as they develop and become more experienced. Of course, like any development, that will happen more easily when an individual wants to develop those skills and characteristics, and in the case of leadership, moral character and personal integrity must underpin the purpose of any change. This corresponds with Lambert's (2002) writing that certain criteria need to exist in effective leadership, for example, a sense of purpose along with ethics, honesty and trust. Lambert also asserts that leaders need to ensure that their egos do not get in the way of effectiveness, a personal issue that we suggest you reflect on in relation to your own leadership, especially if you find yourself in a difficult situation.

## REFLECTION

- Where are you on your leadership learning journey?
- What is your next step going to be? How do you want to develop further?
- How can you use this book to continue that leadership learning journey?

We would urge you to engage with the text and take time out to reflect on how it relates to you and your practice. If you are open to the need for change and growth, we believe you will be even more effective in the future. You also need to be willing to deeply reflect on who you are and what leadership means to you and for what purpose you lead. Once you are clear, you can portray that to others. (Do consider getting support to reflect at this level; many people find they need a leadership coach to ask the right questions and to prevent any personal sabotage to greater personal understanding.)

When exploring what other developments you might pursue as a result of reading this book, you might like to refer to Kelloway and Barling (2010), who provide a comprehensive outline of the effectiveness of leadership development interventions (training and coaching) and their impact on improved perceptions of leadership by staff. Or explore the NHS Leadership Academy and the leadership framework introduced in 2011 (http://www.leadershipacademy.nhs.uk) and the Kings Fund (http://www.kingsfund.org.uk) websites for excellent further reading on current leadership thinking in health care.

In general, we believe that leadership development should have a context-specific focus that allows leaders to make links to their practice to improve service delivery. We also advocate an action research, or implementation and evaluation cycle of improvement, in all aspects of any development to measure the impact of any changes. These elements are quite widely supported in the literature on leadership development (see Piggot-Irvine [2006, 2008] for a summary) and will support any ongoing investment in development.

This book is designed to help you reflect on where you are now to enable you to move forward in your leadership development journey. It does not claim to encompass all knowledge about leadership, but openly and genuinely shares what we have found useful in our own practices over our careers to date. You can read the book from start to finish, rereading it again over time, or you can choose to jump straight in to certain chapters over time to re-evaluate your development in priority areas. Use the book in the way that best suits your own needs and let us know how you get on.

# References

Argyris, C. 1986. Skilled incompetence. *Harvard Business Review* 64 (5): 74–80.

Argyris, C. 1990. *Overcoming organisational defenses: Facilitating organisational learning.* Needham Heights, MA: Allyn and Bacon.

Avolio, B. J., and W. L. Gardner. 2005. Authentic leadership development: Getting to the root of positive forms of leadership. *The Leadership Quarterly* 16: 315–38.

Bolton, R., and D. G. Bolton. 1984. *Social style/management style: Developing productive work relationships.* New York: Amacom.

Cardno, C. 1994. *A reflective model of leadership for organisational learning.* Unpublished paper, UNITEC Institute of Technology, Auckland.

Clarke, N. 2006. Emotional intelligence training: A case of caveat emptor. *Human Resource Development Review* 5: 422–41.

Cummings, G., H. Lee, T. MacGregor, M. Davey, C. Wong, L. Paul, and E. Stafford. 2008. Factors contributing to nursing leadership: A systematic review. *Journal of Health Services Research & Policy* 13 (4): 240–48.

Daft, R. L., and A. Pirola-Merlo. 2009. *The leadership experience: Asia Pacific edition.* South Melbourne, Victoria, Australia: Cengage Learning.

Davidson, S. J. 2010. Complex responsive processes: A new lens for leadership in twenty-first-century health care. *Nursing Forum* 45 (2): 108–17.

Dick, B., and T. Dalmau. 1999. *Values in action: Applying the ideas of Argyris and Schon*, 2nd ed. Chapel Hill, Brisbane: Interchange.

Fein, E. C., C. Vasiliu, and A. Tziner. 2011. Individual values and preferred leadership behaviors: A study of Romanian managers. *Journal of Applied Social Psychology* 41 (2): 515–35.

Goleman, D. 2000. Leadership that gets results. *Harvard Business Review* 78 (2): 78–90.

Goleman, D. 2006. *Social intelligence: The new science of human relationships.* New York: Bantam Dell.

Goleman, D., R. Boyatzis, and A. McKee. 2002. *The new leaders: Transforming the art of leadership into the science of results.* London: Little Brown.

Hersey, P., and K. H. Blanchard. 1977. *Management of organisation behavior: Utilizing human resources*, 3rd ed. Englewood Cliffs, NJ: Prentice-Hall.

Howieson, B., and T. Thiagarajah. 2011. What is clinical leadership? A journal-based meta-review. *The International Journal of Clinical Leadership* 17: 7–18.

Johnson, P., and J. Indvik. 1999. Organisational benefits of having emotionally intelligent managers and employees. *Journal of Workplace Learning* 11 (3): 84–88.

Kelloway, E. K., and J. Barling. 2010. Leadership development as an intervention in occupational health psychology. *Work & Stress* 24 (3): 260–79.

Kings Fund. 2011. *The future of leadership and management in the NHS: No more heroes.* Report from the Kings Fund Commission on Leadership and Management in the NHS. The Kings Fund, London.

Kings Fund. 2012. *Leadership and engagement for improvement in the NHS: Together we can.* Report from the Kings Fund Leadership Review. The Kings Fund, London.

Kouzes, J., and B. Posner. 2002. *The leadership challenge.* San Francisco: Jossey-Bass.

Lambert, L. 2002. Towards a deepened theory of constructivist leadership. In *The constructivist leader*, ed. L. Lambert, D. Walker, D. Zimmerman, J. E. Cooper, M. D. Lambert, M. E. Gardner, and M. Szabo, 34–62. New York: Teachers College Press.

Levy, L. and Bentley, M. 2007. *More Right than Real: The shape of authentic leadership in New Zealand.* Prepared for BDO Spicers.

Meglino, B. M., and E. C. Ravlin. 1998. Individual values in organisations: Concepts, controversies, and research. *Journal of Management* 24: 251–89.

Northouse, P. G. 2004. *Leadership: Theory and practise.* Thousand Oaks, CA: Sage.

Piggot-Irvine, E. 2001. *Appraisal, reducing control: Enhancing effectiveness.* Ph.D. thesis submitted to Massey University, University of New Zealand.

Piggot-Irvine, E. 2006. Establishing criteria for effective professional development and use in evaluating an action research programme. *Journal of In-service Education* 32 (4): 477–96.

Piggot-Irvine, E. 2008. An action research based leadership professional development with depth: Hidden challenges for organisations and facilitators. *Australasian Journal of Business and Social Inquiry* 6 (1): 30–49.

Piggot-Irvine, E. 2012. Creating authentic collaboration: A central feature of effectiveness. In *Action research for sustainable development in a turbulent world*, ed. O. Zuber-Skerritt, 89–107. Bingley, UK: Emerald.

Schaubroeck, J., S. Lam, and S. E. Cha. 2007. Embracing transformational leadership: Team values and the impact of leader behavior on team performance. *Journal of Applied Psychology* 92: 1020–30.

UK Chartered Institute for Personnel and Development. 2012. *Perspectives on leadership in 2012: Implications for HR.* http://www.cipd.co.uk/hr-resources/research/perspectives-leadership-2012.aspx. (For members only)

Welbourne, D., R. Warwick, C. Carnall, and D. Fathers. 2012. *Leadership of whole systems.* London: The Kings Fund.

Williams, S. 2004. *Evidence of the contribution leadership development for professional groups makes in driving their organisations forward.* Prepared for the NHS Modernisation Agency Leadership Centre, Henley Management College, Henley on Thames.

Yukl, G. A. 2002. *Leadership in organisations.* Englewood Cliffs, NJ: Prentice-Hall.

# 2 Practical Leadership in Nursing and Health Care

Daksha Malik, Dee Wilkinson and
Suzanne Henwood

Now that you have looked at some of the key issues in current leadership thinking, this chapter explores how you can apply those concepts to yourself as a leader.

## Understanding Self

One of the greatest attributes of being a great leader is having a deeper understanding of oneself. This includes a higher degree of self-awareness, a recognition and acknowledgement of one's strengths and weaknesses, along with a belief system that supports them—not only in the achievement of one's goals, but also in overcoming the challenges that one may face on a day-to-day basis. The more you know about yourself, your mind, and your behaviours, the greater appreciation and understanding you will have of the people around you. It's much better to work with what you know, rather than what you don't know.

It is widely accepted that the most valuable asset in any organisation is its people. Collins (2001) goes further by stating that it is about having the right people in the right roles that enables the move from good to great. Therefore, investing in getting the most out of yourself and your people is critical for personal and organisational success.

How you think and behave will determine your effectiveness as a 'leader'. It is therefore a useful investment of time to explore the way in which you operate—not only to assess your effectiveness from your external expression of yourself (your communication and behaviours), but also your internal self (thoughts/mind-set and beliefs).

# Communication with Self and Other

If you work on getting the communication right with yourself, then you are far more likely to get your communication right with others. It is completely normal to have an 'internal voice', and how you talk to yourself can have an enormous impact on your ability to function, your well-being and your decision making. This is highlighted particularly when under pressure. There are some various aspects of communication with 'self' that are worth considering further.

## REFLECTION

- Self:
  - Inner voice—is your inner voice critical or encouraging?
  - How do you stay focussed when your mental chatter is getting in the way, or when you are simultaneously juggling a number of tasks?
  - What sort of internal dialogue goes on for you in different situations?
  - How does your emotional state affect your communication?
- Other:
  - How good are you at using silence and stillness to really connect with people in order to allow deeper information to emerge?
  - How courageous are you at giving and receiving feedback?
  - How often are your instructions misinterpreted?
  - What impact have your assumptions and judgements of others made on your ability to make relationships?

Many healthcare professionals choose these particular jobs due to a deep sense of caring for others. However, many are much harder on themselves than they ever would be on their patients. If you were encouraging a patient to start walking after a hip operation, that individual would no doubt be allowed to make mistakes and get things wrong. With encouragement and gentle coercing, you would help boost the patient's confidence and strength, step by step.

Whilst an internal steely attitude to self, such as 'just get on with it', 'stop complaining' and 'you really messed up that time' can indeed galvanise a certain type of forward momentum, this may not be the most resourceful way to get the best results in practice.

Whenever people chastise themselves for a mistake, they are knocking away their own confidence, reaffirming any negative self-belief. This will result in limiting themselves as to what they may be truly capable of, without even realising they are doing it. You cannot expect yourself to grow and develop as effectively as possible, if you mentally beat yourself up every time something goes wrong. Changing a habit of a lifetime can be a challenge, but with persistence and patience (and we suggest the support of a good coach) you can start to run a whole new script that will open up the next level of personal development for yourself.

So what simple, practical steps can you take right now to begin that new way of communicating with yourself? This chapter will help you to slow down and change the mental chatter that may be taking you off focus. As soon as you notice any negative thinking, simply say 'Stop!' or consciously change it to a voice you cannot take seriously (Donald Duck for example) or a positive expression ('I can do this'). Then refocus back to the task in hand. You can also help yourself by eliminating (or at least minimising) any distractions, e.g., close your office door, inform staff that you don't want to be disturbed if at all possible, and give yourself space to focus on the task. Decision making is not most effective when done solely in the head, and you need space and quiet to involve your heart and gut. You also need to learn to trust what you hear and perceive from within.

When you think of your internal voice, talk to yourself as you would a patient or your own best friend. Speak from your adult place (see Chapter 4) with respect, based on evidence and facts. Never underestimate the power of negative, or positive, self-talk for setting the tone for behaviour and success.

## ACTIVITY

To develop greater internal self-respect, begin to notice when you may be speaking negatively to yourself.

- What words or phrases do you commonly use to speak to yourself when things do not go well?

- If you were to replace those words with something more encouraging, what could you say instead and what difference would that make to how you feel?

- Over time we recommend that you practise self-forgiveness and self-encouragement until it comes naturally. This places you in the centre of an ongoing, positive, developmental journey, where you are integral to your own coaching and personal growth.

## Self-Management: Setting the Right Mind-Set

Of course, you need to underpin these changes with a positive self-belief and mind-set. This will give you the confidence to lead. The better you know yourself and trust yourself, the better you will understand why you operate the way you do and what motivates you. In turn, this will help you to better understand the people around you and give you confidence in your actions.

# REFLECTION

- So how well do you really know yourself?

- When did you (or will you) decide that you want to be an even more effective leader, and what motivates you in that decision?

- What do you think about yourself as a leader? (Complete the sentence: As a leader I ____.)

- What are your personal beliefs about yourself and your leadership ability? Do these support you in your role?

- If not, what more positive beliefs will help you?

Take a moment to ask yourself these questions and answer them as openly and honestly as you can. It's easy to give textbook answers or answers that you think you would be expected to give. But we would like to suggest that you invest some time in really opening up and exploring who you are and your true feelings about yourself and your role before moving on to other activities in the book.

## ACTIVITY

To assist you further in exploring where you are now in relation to leadership, we want to share with you a model (Figure 2.1) from Neuro-Linguistic Programming (NLP). (Note: NLP communication is explored in greater depth in Chapter 4.) The model is: Neurological Levels of Change (Dilts and DeLozier 2000), which lends itself very well as an exercise of self-exploration and understanding. Detailed below are some questions from this model that you may find useful. You can work through these yourself or have someone facilitate the exercise for you by asking you the questions (and recording your responses), thereby allowing you to fully immerse yourself in your thoughts. This exercise is also a great vehicle for two-way support between yourself and your peers who also wish to explore leadership development.

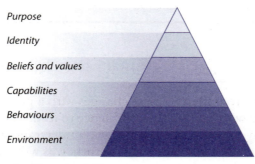

**Figure 2.1:** Neurological Levels of Change.

The levels within the model form the basis of a step-by-step facilitated reflection. Begin at *environment* and work through each level in turn (only moving on when you feel you have fully explored each area).

- *Environment:* Thinking about your current situations, in a range of contexts: where, when and with whom do you lead? Consider location, timing, any external constraints and key people involved. What other areas would you like to lead that you are not leading at the moment?

- *Behaviours:* What do you *do* when you are leading? What are your behaviours? How do others see you behave? Which of your behaviours support your role and which behaviours do you know don't? What do you think others think of your behaviours?

- *Capabilities:* What are your capabilities? What skills and knowledge do you have to be the best leader you can be? Are there any skills or knowledge that are missing that would make you an even better leader? If so, where can you get these?

- *Beliefs and values:* What is important to you about being a leader? What do you care about? What do you believe about yourself as a leader? What do you believe to be true about leadership? What is motivating you? Is there anything that is de-motivating you, and what can you do about this?

- *Identity:* What is your identity as a leader? Who do you see yourself as when you are leading? Who are you when you are leading well? Who are you when you are not leading well?

- *Purpose:* For what purpose are you leading? You may want to consider what's in it for you, for your team, for your department, for your organisation, for your patients, for society or anything else for which you are doing what you are doing (for example, some higher spiritual calling).

At each level, be honest; you have nothing to gain by not answering the questions fully and openly. If you are working with someone else, it can be useful to ask him or her to take notes to give back to you about what you have said.

---

**Tip:** The most effective way to do this exercise is to lay out some cards on the floor, each named with the level on it, and then to physically stand on/ move to each new level to explore what each one means to you. The physical movement will help you to focus on each layer separately and will emphasise a change and/or a new perspective.

You can also return down the levels, noting how actively reflecting on each level may have generated some changes on the return pathway. Look to see that the levels are congruent and aligned throughout and that each supports the other levels.

Having carried out a self-assessment, how confident are you on a scale of 1–10 in your ability to be the most effective leader you can be (where 1 is not confident at all and 10 is totally confident)?

If the score you have given to yourself is less than 10, what do you need to do to get closer to 10?

What needs to happen to get to a 10?

Or if that feels like too big a leap, try going one or two points up the scale. You can do this in stages! Your level of self-confidence will impact on your own performance and how others perceive you. Your self-belief and confidence in your ability to be an effective leader is a cornerstone in your leadership development. Listen to your words, your feelings and be aware of any non-verbal language that might highlight areas that you do not feel completely confident with. If you require assistance with this, consider finding yourself a qualified NLP coach to get the most out of this tool.

## Key Characteristics to Foster in Relation to Self-Awareness and Leading Self

While some people have natural leadership ability, for most of us, leadership skills need to be developed and built over time. This is even more effective if we are mindful and proactive in working on the characteristics that drive the development of these skills.

Many leaders will have had some form of personality profile and/or psychometric testing in order to gain insight into their preferred way of working, their strengths and weaknesses. This is an excellent place to start from, as these can provide some more 'objective' data to consider alongside your personal reflections. But whether or not you have this information to hand, Table 2.1 is a helpful list of some of the core characteristics required to foster leadership development.

All of the information in Table 2.1 comes under the heading of self-management. If you are not looking after yourself, you are far less likely to have the *energy levels* that you need to perform effectively. *On Form* (Loehr and Schwartz 2006–2011, p. 861) describes how to manage energy effectively in order to maintain full engagement in our work and lives. It states: 'According to American data gathered by the Gallup organisation in early 2001, some 55% of staff are disengaged at work'. This is referring to people that are turning up and functioning but are no longer staying focussed. They are no longer fully engaged with tasks or being pro-active and creative in their approach. Conversely, corporate burnout is one of the major challenges that organisations and individuals face. Sadly, a culture has developed where it is seen as a badge of honour to turn up early and leave late. Healthcare professionals in particular have an overwhelming sense of responsibility when it comes to their patients/services. The result is that the majority of people are putting in excessive hours and

**Table 2.1:** Core Characteristics of Leadership Development

| Reflection | Do you keep a reflective journal? How do you factor in reflection to your practice and then stay mindful of the outcomes? Do you share your reflections with others (peer, mentor, coach) to further enhance the value of that reflection? |
|---|---|
| Self-discipline | What strategies do you have in place to keep yourself to task, stay focussed and see things through? |
| Self-awareness | Are you able to effectively receive feedback in a non-defensive way? Do you notice what makes you react and also how you impact others on an emotional level? Do you know what drives you and how to maximise your efforts? |
| Self-management | How do you ensure that you take care of yourself (physically, mentally, emotionally and spiritually)? How are your energy levels? How will you avoid burnout? What do you need to factor in to maintain a healthy work/life balance? |
| Communication | How do you practise being articulate in your language in order to maintain rapport and respect? Is your communication clear? Do you encourage others to check out communication with you to minimise misunderstandings? |
| Empathy | Can you genuinely feel what it is like for others? What is the difference between sympathy and empathy, and how might each affect your leadership? |
| Courage and resilience | How are you developing your skill of courage to do the right thing? How do you keep moving forward, even when up against obstacles? Are you able to manage conflict effectively? What might stop you having the conversations you know you need to have? |
| Authenticity | How do you manage to honour your values in alignment with the organisation's if/when they differ? Do you think you are genuine and authentic, and how do you know? Would your colleagues be able to voice what is important to you? |
| Ego management | Are your decisions based on the greater good or your own benefit or promotion? Can you admit when you are wrong and apologise? Can you actively flex your leadership style to meet changing demands and needs? How would your peers answer these questions about you? |
| Vision | Do you have a clear vision and direction with which to inspire and motivate followers? Can you keep sight of the strategic overview whilst being mindful of the here and now? How quickly and accurately can you gain and voice a useful perspective? |

increasingly feel overwhelmed and exhausted by their work. At some level, both the organisation and the individual need to start to take responsibility for changing this culture, as it is detrimental to both individual and organisational effectiveness.

*On Form* (Loehr and Schwartz 2006–2011) goes on to say that it has been proven in all fields that rest and recovery are essential for peak performance. An athlete normally trains around 90% of the time to enable them to perform at their peak for the other 10% of their time. Athletes also are likely to have a few months off a year to recover and rest. However, in the corporate (and healthcare) world, it is likely that as leader you are expected to perform at your peak for around 90% of the time, with maybe 10% of time to recover and rest during annual leave. Sadly, even then people find it hard, often not taking leave, and when they do, they often find it difficult to disengage from their work, still continuing to check e-mails, etc., on portable devices.

As a leader it is essential that you adopt a healthy approach to work-life balance for both yourself and staff. Life has a natural ebb and flow, but there is now a great risk that we, as human beings, have fallen into the trap of thinking we can override this. Peak performance, greater productivity and innovative thinking can only happen when people have the *energy* to fully engage and focus.

Loehr and Schwartz (2006–2011, p. 861) define four key areas of energy that are inextricably linked (see Table 2.2). They all need to be addressed in order for peak performance to occur.

Suggestions for putting this into practice:

- Take a short break every 90 minutes (even if it is just a 10-minute break to stretch your legs or to rehydrate).

- Eat something healthy every 2 hours to maintain energy levels.

- Drink plenty of water and cut down on caffeine.

**Table 2.2:** Four Key Energy Areas

| Physical | Emotional | Mental | Spiritual |
|---|---|---|---|
| Sleeping – 7 hours | Feelings | Focus | Purpose greater than yourself |
| Eating healthily | Relationship | Thinking skills | Values |
| Drinking – water intake | Processing/ reflection | Mental preparation | Goals |
| Physical fitness | Empathy | Time management | Commitment |
| Breathing properly | Forgiveness | Completing tasks | Enthusiasm |
| | Dealing with stress | | |
| | Emotional management | | |

- Address any negative thoughts and feelings, as these will drain your energy.

- Gain clarity on your purpose and maintain your focus on that.

- Take regular exercise (ideally at least 20 minutes a day to raise your heart rate) and avoid sitting for long periods of time.

- Be honest with yourself and others.

- Build courage to resolve any conflicts. This avoids holding onto negativity over time.

## REFLECTION

- How would you rate your overall sense of well-being against these criteria?

- What area could you improve on? And how? When will you introduce that into your new routine?

## Emotional and Social Intelligence

Another area important to self-awareness is emotional and social intelligence, popularised by Daniel Goleman and discussed in Chapter 1:

> Emotional intelligence includes self-awareness and impulse control, persistence, zeal and motivation, empathy and social deftness. These are qualities that mark people who excel: whose relationships flourish, who are stars in the workplace. (Goleman 1996, back cover)

The term *emotional intelligence* is subject to many definitions. With respect to leadership, we would like to define it as the ability to determine what is emotionally going on for 'ourselves and others' and understanding why.

Many leaders can be academically intelligent, but lack the skills of emotionally connecting their feelings to themselves or others: They do not engage their heart in decision making or relationships. For example, if leaders don't have the awareness to identify their own emotions, they could easily ignore them. The feelings are then more likely to be 'acted out' in behaviour (especially when under pressure) and having an impact on others' feelings, which they may not then be aware of, creating a potentially negative cycle of responses.

We know that people in general will give more, be more loyal and perform better if they feel valued and cared about. This comes from a belief that there is a genuine emotional connection with them. As leaders, the more skilful and developed we become at noticing what is going on for others and for ourselves, the greater will be the speed and depth of connection, which opens up the potential for effective relationships and improved performance.

## REFLECTION

Think of people you have spent time with. What are you noticing at an emotional and physical level when you are communicating with (a) someone you relate well to and (b) someone who appears more difficult to work with?

Thinking of yourself:

- What type of person creates a particular type of feeling/reaction in you?
- Do you understand why you are feeling these feelings?
- What behavioural impact does that have on you?
- What strategies can you create to manage your emotions more effectively?

Thinking of others:

- What is happening, on an emotional level, to the person you are communicating with?
- What might they be feeling as a result of any interaction with you?
- What clues can you gain from their body language?
- What impact have you had on them?

In general, the level of emotional intelligence in people can be described as follows:

- *Little emotional intelligence*: May not even notice what impact they have had on others
- *Some emotional intelligence*: May notice at a subconscious level but not connect consciously with this awareness
- *High emotional intelligence*: Will not only notice the impact, but will also give time and space and use appropriate questions (in a non-judgemental way) to check out any perceived impact to ensure that the most appropriate action is taken

Rock (2006, p. 177) states: 'Another reason for checking on people's emotions early in the conversation is to address any strong emotions that might get in the way of useful conversations'. This takes courage and openness, which may also raise issues of vulnerability, but it is a starting point for effective communication and influence.

It has been found that much of our communication is based on our body language and tone of voice, not just the actual words spoken. Therefore, developing sensitivity to 'noticing' is key to good communication. At very subtle levels, people reflect their feelings in their body language, regardless of what is being said. Someone might say they are feeling fine, when actually their body language, tone of voice and/or facial expressions, are not congruent with their words.

Imagine a patient who is finding it difficult to talk. How do you know what that person's needs are? What clues are you picking up from this individual? Equally with staff, it is often easy to ignore emotional cues when we are under pressure or not sure how to deal with something.

For example:

*Practise noticing in others*

- Do you notice the degree of skin reddening change?
- Do people look away in a certain direction?
- Do their pupils dilate or constrict?
- Can they hold eye contact?
- Do their lips tighten or go thin?
- Does their breathing quicken?
- Does their voice change pitch?
- Do they fidget or look uncomfortable?

**Note:** Having begun to notice, you will then have to explore what those changes mean for that individual. Do not assume you know what the changes mean, or that changes mean the same thing in different people.

*Notice body language and really listen to the whole person*

Body language is a constant source of communication and will often be communicating what is *not* being said. Very often, staff, peers and employees will bring issues to their manager but lack the confidence to be really honest about what is going on for them. People by and large need to feel really safe, both physically and emotionally, before they can connect and communicate in a meaningful way. This brings us right back to the need for a good relationship, built on trust, to encourage open and honest communication. Noticing any signs of incongruence between what is said and what someone's body language is saying is often a cue to use enquiring questions to get to the real issue. However, do not assume that you know what any apparent incongruence means. Moving on to 'mind reading' can be disastrous. Use your noticing skills to explore meanings with each individual to ensure clarity and openness between you.

Another skill worth developing is listening at a 'global' level. While hearing the words, practise keeping your own thoughts and judgements out of the equation; pause your own conversation (internally and externally) to genuinely listen to the other person before bringing your own perspective into the mix (listen and observe and withhold any judgement). Use culturally appropriate eye contact (or not) to build rapport, and use the previously discussed noticing skills to prompt further questions to assist clarity. Be aware of your own feelings, which can inadvertently be projected onto the person you are listening to.

## REFLECTION

Find someone willing to explore this with you. Start to really notice what is happening physically for the other person you are communicating with as you discuss an agreed topic. Explore with them what was happening and what any changes you noticed meant for them.

## TOOL

### The Emotional Bank Account

An effective leader is genuinely interested in staff/colleagues on a personal level. This can be as simple as taking time to enquire how somebody is or how his or her weekend went (whilst being authentic). People will see right through any approach which does not show you genuinely care or are interested. Try to remember some specific details in regard to colleagues so that you can show you were listening next time you talk, to show genuine interest. Some of the more direct, reserved or introverted leaders may see involving themselves in such small talk as a waste of time. However, the opposite is true.

Each time you show a genuine, positive desire to connect and remember what may be important to another person, a deposit is made into the emotional bank account. With the emotional bank account full, it is there for when a withdrawal may be needed. For example, there may be a space in rota to fill and you need a staff member to work an hour's overtime or an extra shift. With a full emotional bank account, the likelihood of engagement and reciprocation is high. It could be argued that this could be seen as manipulative, but as long as the communication is genuine and authentic on the leader's part, this needn't be the case. Just check internally that the intention behind your actions has no manipulative or self-serving component.

# Power and Assertiveness

Power and assertiveness are two more areas we will briefly explore in relation to working with and influencing others.

## REFLECTION

- What do we mean when we talk about power and assertiveness in leadership, and why is it important?

- How do we ensure it is appropriate and positive?

- At what point in our conversations can we utilise power to gain a the outcomes we are looking for, and when do we need to be more assertive in leadership?

- How is this seen within a collaborative team, where different people may have different, strongly held views about what needs to happen?

The definition of *assert*, according to the Collins English Dictionary, is to '**compel** recognition of one's individuality, authority or rights. Self-confident and firm in dealing with others and getting one's way'.

Healthcare professionals can find it difficult to be as assertive as they need to be, due to their caring nature and a long history of hierarchy in practice. Some individuals in caring professions can be so concerned for another's well-being that they may put their own/organisational needs aside to avoid the risk of offending or upsetting others, thereby slipping into passive behaviours. This can then result in their work burden increasing, their time being further stretched and their own well-being impacted. This can also have a detrimental effect on service delivery, while others are keen to dominate and push their own views forward.

Paradoxically, when you are able to be assertive, you are often treated with greater respect. People appreciate knowing where they stand. When you express your needs respectfully, it enables others to be clearer in how they respond.

One popular model of communication outlines three ways of communicating that have been classed as *passive*, *assertive* and *aggressive* (with assertive being advocated as the most appropriate to gain influence in a professional setting). If you, as an individual have suffered from low self-confidence or self-esteem, you may find that stepping up to being more assertive actually feels like you are being aggressive. But assertiveness is about balance. It is about recognising what needs to be done and respecting your own and others' rights. It is about acting fairly, with empathy, and again being aware of your intentions.

The greater understanding you have of who you are and the greater belief you have in the value you bring, the easier it will be to be assertive. The ability to be assertive is linked to where you are in terms of self-esteem, self-confidence and self-worth.

Being able to be assertive can also lower your stress levels. You know you have your own personal power, so therefore you are less likely to feel threatened or victimised when things don't go your way, or as you had planned.

Being assertive is about good communication and feeling confident in what you say, when spoken from the 'adult' place (Chapter 4). Table 2.3 compares the three approaches.

## REFLECTION

- At what times in your role is it important to be more assertive?
- What areas of assertiveness do you need to improve in?
- Do you communicate mostly from the middle column of Table 2.3, and if not, what do you need to do differently?
- How can you safely practise being assertive so it feels more natural in practice?

**Table 2.3:** Passive, Assertive and Aggressive Communication

| Passive | Assertive | Aggressive |
|---|---|---|
| **General attitude** | **General attitude** | **General attitude** |
| Submissive | Optimistic | Attacking |
| Long-suffering | Positive | Impatient |
| Self-blaming | Respectful | Blaming |
| Deferent | Fair | Dominant |
| | Compromising | Hurtful |
| | | Single-minded |
| **Words used** | **Words used** | **Words used** |
| Sorry | I appreciate | You will |
| Would you mind? | I would like | Make sure you do |
| If you like | I feel | Should |
| It's only me | I don't like | I told you so |
| I don't mind | How can we resolve this? | I don't care |
| **Body language** | **Body language** | **Body language** |
| Fidgety | Relaxed | Clenched fists |
| Shuffling | Upright | Finger pointing |
| Eyes down | Eye contact | Folded arms |
| Soft-spoken | Clear, audible voice | Staring |
| Mumbling | | Stiff |
| | | Leaning towards |

*Note:* This table was developed by Stella Gardener.

**Note:** There is a risk that if you are too direct in your communication, you can come across as aggressive. This is likely to happen when you are communicating your needs and not listening to, or understanding, the other's perspective. Being aggressive often comes with impatience, the need to control or feeling disempowered, and it shows in confrontational body language and a raised voice. Knowing this can help you to choose to communicate assertively.

## Power in Relation to Leadership

Many leaders are naturally perceived to be powerful and may possess a great deal of power due to their position. Leadership and power can be closely related. For example, leaders will potentially have the power to recruit, to manage performance and to discipline their staff. They can be in charge of whether you are promoted or demoted, get the leave you request or are supported in professional development. This alone can create dynamics in relationships that, if not managed appropriately, can be damaging and abusive.

John French and Bertram Raven (1959) are two social psychologists who conducted a notable study to understand what *power* means in leadership. They identified five power bases that people operate from.

1. *Legitimate*: The person (due to their role) has the right to make demands and to expect compliance and obedience from others.

2. *Reward*: This derives from one person's ability to compensate another for compliance.

3. *Expert*: This is based on a person's superior skill and knowledge.

4. *Referent*: This is the result of a person's perceived attractiveness, worthiness, and right to respect from others.

5. *Coercive*: This comes from a belief that a person can punish others for non-compliance.

By understanding more about these power bases, you can begin to reflect on your own style. Consider how these styles may have changed over time, for example with legitimate power being appropriate in previous hierarchical structures, but maybe less so in modern collaborative leadership styles. The most effective leaders use mainly referent and expert power. Basically, they are respected for their superior knowledge and worthiness as a leader, regardless of the organisational style they work within. Gaining respect then, and having a strong belief in your judgement are key areas for effective leadership.

## REFLECTION

Take time to think about which power base you are more likely to use. How can you develop the more effective areas of *referent* and *expert* power into your leadership style so that you have a positive influence on your colleagues, team and organisation?

Power, influence and leadership all need to be considered when reflecting on your own practice. Key to all three, we believe, is you being aware of your intentions in each area, ensuring you act from a position of honesty and integrity in relationship with others and constantly reflecting on your behaviours and others to ensure that your drive to change is positively motivated, ethical and professional in implementation.

## REFLECTION

Before moving on, what is it that drives you? For what purpose? What is your highest motivation to change?

Keep the answers visible to guide your desired future. The next chapter will help you to explore your professional vision in more depth.

# Personality Types and Individual Difference in Communications, Learning, Being and Leading

Taking the time to really understand yourself is the first major step to understanding others. You can't lead effectively if you don't understand people or if you are unable to communicate, to build relationships, to influence or to inspire. A successful leader is one that people want to follow. A leader with no followers is merely a person going for a walk on their own.

The way that you operate, function, process, think and behave is a product of your experiences in life and of the environments to which you have been exposed in your life. Therefore, as no two people in the world have lived identical lives, it is fair to say that each and every one of us is unique. Whilst uniqueness is to be embraced and celebrated, it can create barriers to understanding other people.

At a subconscious level, it is easy to assume that the people around you think the way that you do, value the things that you value, process information the way that you process because these are ways that you know work for you. And let's face it, it's where things are familiar, where you are comfortable, where you feel safe and in control. Interestingly, though, we learn and develop at the boundaries of our comfort zone, so being more comfortable to push those boundaries out and to broaden your perspectives is a good thing.

In reality, you soon learn that people have their own minds and interpretations, their own values, their own interests and their own goals and agendas, all of which may be similar to yours or not, and this makes your interactions a little more complex. Assuming similarity can lead to misinterpretation of the motivations and behaviours of the people around you whose minds operate differently to your own.

Successful leaders of today value differences in people and welcome individuality and uniqueness, as these are all attributes that bring with them new and fresh ways of thinking and support evolution and progress. Leaders value attributes that challenge the norm, push the boundaries and bring about change, and they work to see how each person can contribute to the whole, embracing the difference and diversity of real life in a global society. Organisations no longer want leaders who produce clones of themselves, people who all think the same, people who all agree with them and people who conform just because they feel pressured to do so and because it's easier to. Today's leaders take on board the fact that there are no right or wrong ways of thinking—there are just different ways of thinking. It's about finding new ways of working that can push boundaries whilst still working safely and within the constraints of regulatory and moral ethics. It is only when this mind-set is truly adopted that you can begin to work even more effectively with the people around you through being open to and respecting thoughts and ways that are different to yours. Making this type of shift in mind-set may not happen overnight and will require effort and commitment along with a strong desire to see long-term change. It takes courage and true leadership by strong, effective leaders who clearly know who they are, what they stand for and where they are going. A leader must have a good relationship with the team so that the team follows or, better still, drives forward the changes themselves due to the leader's actions.

The ability to recognise, respect and work with differences is an important aspect of any leadership role. Whilst others around you may operate differently to you, this doesn't necessarily mean that they are less (or more) effective than you. Differences can and do exist in all aspects of leadership, from communication and decision making to problem solving and planning. Effective leaders will have sufficient behavioural flexibility in themselves to be able to adapt and work with people who think and operate, sometimes, very differently to themselves. As an effective leader, you will support the people around you to operate to their optimum, providing clear direction whilst giving each of them the responsibility to deliver results. To do this you truly need to understand yourself, and this chapter has hopefully begun to encourage and enable you to increase and improve your self-awareness and to open up awareness of wider leadership effectiveness.

## References

Collins, J. 2001. *Good to great: Why some companies make the leap and others don't*. Random House, London.

Dilts, R., and J. DeLozier. 2000. Logical levels. *Encyclopaedia of NLP*. NLP University press. http://nlpuniversitypress.com/html2/LmLz38.html.

French, J. R. P., and B. Raven. 1959. The bases of social power. In *Group dynamics*, ed. D. Cartwright and A. Zander. New York: Harper & Row.

Goleman, D. 1996. *Emotional intelligence*. London: Bloomsbury.

Loehr, J., and T. Schwartz. 2006–2011. *On form*. London: Nicholas Brealey.

Rock, D. 2006. *Quiet leadership: Six steps to transforming performance at work*. New York: Harper Collins.

References

# 3 Understanding Self: Creating Your Vision

Karen Moxom and Donna Blinston

## Leadership

There has long been an argument as to whether a leader is born or created. Riggio (2009) surmised that one-third of leaders are born and two-thirds are made. What is clear is that leadership is a complex process requiring the leader to be open to and embrace change; to have excellent interpersonal skills, especially in the area of communication; and to have the ability to develop and inspire a vision with the intention of positive social/contextual gain while valuing what is important to the team in order to motivate and develop them to fully contribute and add value.

In this chapter we will explore the importance of understanding your new enhanced self-awareness as a leader and encourage you to use that to create a vision that inspires you and that you can use to inspire others.

## Let's Start with Personal Values

Everyone has personal values, whether or not they are explicitly aware of them. Our values underpin so many of the judgements we make and the actions we take, forming our deep, unconscious belief system representing what is important to us. By understanding our value system, and how it relates to other aspects of our life, we can identify what motivates us and use that to be even more effective at what we do.

One role of values is to create 'boundaries' which we will not cross. More importantly, we will be affected emotionally if these boundaries are crossed by other people we come into contact with, whether they are in our team, our patients, clients, suppliers or other leaders.

Understanding the huge role that values play in our lives means we can better understand their impact on us as individuals, adding another element to our 'self knowing'. We looked briefly at values in Chapter 2 as part of the Neurological Levels Model (Dilts and DeLozier 2000). In reviewing that model, you can see the significance values have to play in influencing our behaviours. The model can be applied to you as an individual or to your team, department or organisation, and you can use it again in this chapter to check that your vision is congruent and well supported across all of the levels represented.

Exploring your values contributes to a deeper sense of self-knowing, which is essential before you can relate to others. We know that as a leader, a big part of your role involves relating to others as well as self, so we will briefly explore three ways of relating to others, using:

- Values
- Metaprograms
- Perceptual positions

## Relating to Others Using Values

As a leader, as well as being aware of your own values, it is important to also be aware of the values of the individuals within your team, and also the values of your organisation. It is likely the values of the organisation underpin their vision, and ideally, these values will ripple down and be reflected in departments, teams and individuals. Of course, the values of individuals can also help to shape the values of the team, the department and the organisation. Ideally, the individual and organisational values will be congruent, with a good match between the espoused values (what people say is important) and actual values (which drive behaviour in practice).

Part of our role, as leaders, is to 'manage' the values of our team and the organisation. We 'manage' because:

- Incongruence within an individual's logical levels (i.e., where the levels do not support each other) can lead to inner conflict and confusion and reduce personal effectiveness.

  Imagine how hard it must be for a drug addict who wants to kick the habit but then has to share a physical environment with other drug users. This environment is in direct conflict with the behaviours the would-be ex-addict would like to exhibit—and goodness knows how this is going to affect that individual's ability to actually come off drugs, especially if the person's own values, such as self-esteem, are not as strong as they could be.

- Differences in values can also lead to conflict or dissatisfaction within a team or organisation.

Have you ever found yourself in a situation where a colleague, supplier or patient says something, and you experience some sort of inner discomfort? You may find yourself wanting to react to their comments verbally, or inwardly mulling over their words and feeling any number of mixed emotions. You may even feel that your inward reaction seems to be disproportionate to the original trigger, which may, to the speaker, have been a simple throwaway comment. These emotional reactions may be caused because something they said is in conflict with something you believe. It may even feel like someone has pushed one of your 'hot buttons'! Your deeply held values have been challenged in some way, and this is called a values conflict.

The important thing to recognise in these situations is what is happening for you or for the other person in your team who is experiencing this reaction. Once there is an understanding that the emotional reaction (or overreaction) is being caused by values being challenged, there are then ways this can be overcome so the conflict can be resolved, rather than be left to potentially fester and eventually affect good working relationships. By having this understanding and awareness, you are able to demonstrate greater self-control in challenging situations and hold on to your emotions (self-management and emotional intelligence are discussed in Chapter 2), rather than just reacting in a potentially negative way.

So how can values conflicts/challenges be resolved?

Sometimes, just acknowledging that there has been a challenge to values in a particular relationship is enough. This will enable persons who have experienced the emotional reaction to logically reason with themselves and understand what has caused the reaction—and then move on.

**CASE STUDY**

For example, a patient died following a sudden unexpected heart attack. The relatives had been called, but it was going to take them 4 hours to get to the hospital. Therefore, the body was on the ward waiting for the relatives to arrive. This was causing the manager concern, as the hospital was on red alert. A member of the staff was completely disgusted by the manager's request to transfer the body to the mortuary.

The emotional response that arose from the staff member was due to her values being challenged because they were both working and looking at the patient's death from different perspectives. However, both parties had an awareness of values, and they were quickly able to recognise that there may have been a values conflict due to different values and priorities. The staff member had personally experienced death recently and wanted

continued ...

to provide the family with the opportunity to say goodbye on the ward, supporting the family's grieving process. The manager, whilst respecting her employee's recent loss, knew that from an organisational perspective, the dead body was blocking a bed of a patient in need of medical attention. One of their key organisational values was to 'provide accessible health care' to everyone who required it. Transferring the dead body to the mortuary would ensure that she was fulfilling that value and support A&E (accident and emergency) through the red alert state of emergency that they were currently experiencing.

The manager spoke with the staff member to find out what the family knew of the patient's condition and whether the patient dying would be a total shock to them. Although the death was sudden and unexpected, the patient had a terminal cancer. Due to this, the manager explained the bed situation and asked the staff member if she would be happy to speak to the chapel of rest, explain the situation, and ask the mortician if he would prepare the body for viewing with the staff member's help. Then, when the family arrived, the staff member could spend that time explaining the events that led to the sudden death of their relative, and then take them to the chapel of rest. This would be more private for the relatives than a curtain around a bed space and would give them time to be together as a family. The manager was respecting the staff member's values and supporting A&E in their red alert state.

By being able to recognise the deeper emotional response which had arisen due to values being challenged (rather than just the surface issue of 'beds'), the manager and staff member were able to negotiate their way around the issue by recognising that there was an even bigger value upon which they could both agree, which was keeping the patient at the heart of the solution.

Awareness of values also provides an excellent framework when performing a personal appraisal/performance review. Values elicitation will transform the appraisal process, providing staff with a sense of clarity, purpose, focus and motivation, not to mention showing genuine interest in them. Identifying what is important to patients, teams and staff enables you to relate to them even more effectively, improve your rapport and make them feel better understood and valued.

However, values are not the only factor. Another useful framework is the 'metaprogram' framework, also from Neuro-Linguistic Programming (NLP). (Note: NLP communication is explored in greater depth in Chapter 4.)

## Relating to Others Using Metaprograms

Have you ever wondered why some people appear to be so different to yourself? How you can find it difficult to understand and relate to them? This is completely normal and true to life, because we are all different!

Everybody filters information they receive differently, distorting, deleting and generalising it, depending on their unique set of filters (see Chapter 4).

Metaprograms determine ways of working, and they act as one of the filters through which information is deleted, distorted or generalised. They work on a similar premise to the work done by Myers (2000), who developed the well-known psychological assessment tool based on the work of Jung in 1971.

Metaprograms recognise that the language we use is interpreted differently, depending on our preferred ways of working. By recognising our own preferences, and those of others, we can use our language to communicate more effectively and motivate our patients, colleagues, teams and ourselves even more effectively.

Metaprograms indicate our preferred patterns of behaviour, which influence how we respond to certain things across different contexts and how we are motivated to act. Each metaprogram has a spectrum, and you could find you are totally one end (X) or the other (Y), mainly X or Y, or equally X and Y.

Metaprograms include: 'towards or away from motivation'; 'introvert or extrovert'; 'big picture or details orientated'; 'options or process driven'; 'matching or mismatching'; 'inferential and literal speaking and listening'; and 'pessimist or optimist'.

Let us explore one of the many useful metaprograms in more depth to both understand ourselves and others: The 'direction' filter—are you motivated *towards* what you want, or *away from* what you do not want? In other words, do you respond better to the carrot or the stick?

'Towards-motivated' people do things because they want to achieve certain outcomes/goals/things. They are good at prioritising and can become oblivious to things going wrong: If you are a 'towards-motivated' individual, you use words such as: *attain*, *get*, *target*, *goal*, *objective*, *obtain*, and *target date*.

An example of a towards statement: 'Through identifying which patients are delayed discharges, we will be able to plan the patient flow through the hospital, freeing up beds on the ward. This will ensure that we achieve the ward's targets and decrease the outpatient waiting list for elective procedures.'

'Away from-motivated' people do things for the opposite reason: They want to avoid certain situations/consequences. They often have trouble focusing on goals because they are easily distracted by things which could go wrong. If you are an 'away from-motivated' person, you use words such as: *avoid*, *steer clear of*, *not have*, *get rid of*, *exclude*, *reduce problems* and *liabilities* and *deadline*.

An example of an away-from statement: 'Identifying which patients are delayed discharges reduces the patient's length of stay in hospital and avoids bed blocking. This will ensure that we decrease the outpatient waiting list for elective procedures, steering us clear away from any liabilities.'

## REFLECTION

Which example statement would motivate you more: towards or away from?

Understanding your own preferred metaprograms allows you to interpret your reactions and behaviour more effectively, especially when communicating with those who fall differently within the spectrum (who you may in the past have just assumed were wrong!). Metaprograms are a valuable leadership tool, as they enable you to understand, predict and influence behaviour through understanding and respecting difference. Where you do not know the staff you are talking to well, by deliberately using a mixture of both language patterns you can ensure that you motivate the whole team, thus boosting team engagement and morale and creating a sense of purpose and direction regardless of their preferences.

An example of using both language spectrums: 'Identifying which patients are delayed discharges reduces the patient's length of stay in hospital and avoids bed blocking. This will ensure that we achieve the ward's targets and decrease the outpatient waiting list for elective procedures.'

We would thoroughly recommend you read Shelle Rose Charvet's (1997) excellent book *Words That Change Minds* to explore the full range of metaprograms and the language patterns associated with them.

# Relating to Others Using Perceptual Positions

The ability to see things from another point of view is another key skill in understanding and relating to other people. It plays an important part in relationship building, negotiations and conflict resolution, as well as allowing us to see the wider picture and thus take a more strategic view of any situation.

Perceptual positions (Dilts and DeLozier 2000) is an NLP technique with various uses, and one of these is to allow us to engage with the NLP presupposition 'respect the other person's model of the world'. By stepping into another person's shoes, you gain insight into their model of the world and a better understanding of their point of view. This can be a really useful tool, especially when relating to the wider, strategic view held by the organisation and ensuring that this is understood by you and your team.

Perceptual positions is a technique which is used to take the emotional charge out of a situation, enabling you to gain multiple perspectives and therefore a greater understanding of any situation.

When used in conflict resolution, perceptual positions has three primary positions: Position 1 is you as you, fully associated into the problem or situation (seeing it through your own eyes). Position 2 is seeing it as the other person in the situation, as if through their eyes. Position 3 is a neutral position, someone who is completely independent, the 'wise old owl' (dissociated, or looking from the outside of the situation—seeing yourself in the picture). Starting in position 1, look at the situation from your perspective. What do you feel from here? Then physically move to position 2, walking away from your perspective, and put yourself in the other person's shoes, looking at the situation from their perspective. What do they see and feel? Move to position 3, in another location, looking over both parties and identify what insights and advice you could now offer, having seen both perspectives and stepped back from the situation. What can you see that they cannot see from this position? What advice would you give yourself now?

You can also add in a fourth position: that of the wider field or system. Looking in on the situation, what does the system see, feel and hear? This is particularly useful within a leadership context, enabling you to gain not only multiple, but also a wider, systems perspective.

Perceptual positioning can be an incredibly powerful technique, and we recommend that you set time aside to walk through it with someone else, maybe even an NLP coach, to gain maximum value from it. Before you read on, decide whom you would like to run through the tool with and contact that person now to set a time and place where you can both explore and benefit from the technique.

## Developing a Mind-Set for Success

We have spoken about understanding self and understanding others, which forms the foundation of relational leadership. Another key to success is having the right mind-set. Developing a mind-set for success will enable you to achieve success even more easily and will also create a culture where your positive attitude becomes infectious to others.

We believe there are six key principles that are required to achieve a mind-set for success:

1. Have a clear vision

2. Build rapport with your team

3. Implement a flexible attitude

4. Take effective action

5. Maintain a resourceful state

6. Embrace the presuppositions of NLP (see ANLP.org.uk for a full list of presuppositions, which, if taken as true, lead to empowering you in your leadership success)

## Have a Clear Vision

Having a clear vision and well-defined outcomes sets up a direction of travel and enables you to stay focussed and achieve your goals. After all, if you don't know where you are going, then how will you know what path to take or how will you realise when you get there? More importantly, if you don't know where you are going, then how can you guide, enthuse and lead your team?

By sharing this vision and staying focussed on the well-defined outcomes, each member of the team will probably have an enhanced sense of purpose and teamwork and will be much more likely to be fully engaged, working with you to achieve your goal.

## Build Rapport with Your Team

Richard Bandler and John Grinder (1979), co-founders of NLP, define rapport as 'demonstrating understanding of the other person's model of the world'. Ellerton (2010, p. 65) explains this further, stating that

> rapport is the basis of any meaningful interaction between two or more people, that rapport is about establishing an environment of trust, understanding, respect and safety which gives a person the freedom to fully express their ideas and concerns and to know that they will be respected by the other person.

Thus rapport is the ability to relate to another in a way that creates a climate of trust and understanding. It is the capability to see each other's point of view and to appreciate each other's feelings, enabling you to lead and your colleagues to follow—or vice versa, in the case of distributed leadership, where roles will change over time, and you may be both leader and follower as you work with different teams and on different projects. Rapport is a central pillar in relational leadership. It begins with a genuine interest in the other person and a desire to really connect with and understand them, in order to allow them to maximise their input whilst still maintaining focus on the goals you have set.

## Implement a Flexible Attitude

By implementing behavioural flexibility, you are better able to adapt to changes. If what you are doing isn't working as well as you would like, you can choose to do something else. Being flexible in your behaviour gives you more choices and many ways to achieve your outcome. Be determined to do whatever it takes (within your values framework) to achieve success, and if something is not working, evaluate why not and be prepared to do it differently. As healthcare practitioners in the twenty-first century, we need to ensure that we are able to adapt our own capabilities and behaviours to reflect the advancements in technology and science while working within the resource constraints that exist worldwide. Health care is changing at a rapid rate: If it is not a new benchmark or governmental target, then it is a new local policy or procedure. On top of these changes, there are multiple research programmes and pharmaceutical developments that are designed to enhance best practice. In addition, role boundaries are shifting, challenging established ways of working. Flexibility and self-awareness equip us with the resources we need to ensure ongoing excellence in patient care.

## Take Effective Action

Without action there are no results, however well formed your outcome may be! Change is always a potential obstacle for everyone; some people will be more comfortable with change than others. However, if you respect and understand what is important to your team and patients (their values), use language that motivates them (metaprograms), take responsibility for the outcome (not blaming others), share your vision with enthusiasm and passion, and respectfully acknowledge and consider any objections, you have a better chance of leading your team to success.

## Stay in a Resourceful State

One of the most powerful ways of achieving a mind-set for success is by developing self-responsibility, both personally and within your team. For you as a leader, this is about recognising that 'the buck stops here' and, therefore, whatever happens within your team or organisation or your sphere of influence, it is ultimately your responsibility.

However, this doesn't mean that everyone else in the organisation can sit back and leave it all to you—far from it. Part of your responsibility as the leader is to empower your team to also take full responsibility for their actions. Imagine how much more powerful and effective your team will be when *every* member is taking 100% responsibility for being fully engaged.

Remember, in any situation, that every person has a choice over how they respond. They can make excuses and blame others so that any possible solutions will need to be the responsibility of other people. This response means they are powerless, making it appear like there is nothing they can do. Or they can take responsibility for the situation, asking appropriate questions in an environment of trust and openness, and be part of the solution. This attitude will empower you as the leader and also empower each individual within your team, as well as developing a culture of respect and self-awareness focussed on continuous improvement.

In NLP, this is known as 'cause and effect', and individuals are said to be 'at cause' when taking responsibility, rather than being affected by everyone and everything else outside their control. Of course, there are situations which will be outside of your control, and even then, you and your team can choose how you respond to those situations, thereby changing any impact on you.

## Embrace the Presuppositions of NLP

The presuppositions of NLP (ANLP.org.uk) are incredibly valuable when it comes to adopting a mind-set for success. The principles which form the foundation of NLP have been modelled from key people who consistently produced superb results, as well as from systems theory and natural laws.

As well as a set of powerful skills, NLP is a philosophy and an attitude that is useful when your goal is excellence in whatever you do.

Discover what happens if you simply act 'as if' the following statements (just three of the presuppositions) are true and adopt these attitudes in your own relationships as a leader, or with patients, other staff and suppliers.

## There Is No Failure, Only Feedback

What seemed like failure can be thought of as success that just stopped too soon. With this understanding, we can stop blaming ourselves and others, find solutions and improve the quality of what we do. After all, how many times did Edison 'fail' in his dream to invent the lightbulb before he actually succeeded?

**Tip:** One of the most valuable ways you can improve your own interactions is by accepting feedback as free consultancy advice and being grateful for the opportunity to make positive changes when the feedback is valid and credible.

### REFLECTION

- How do you generally respond when offered feedback?
- How could you get even more value by reflecting on feedback differently?

## *You Cannot Not Communicate*

Everything about you—your appearance, your voice and your actions—communicates something about you and your organisation all the time. In fact, according to research by Mehrabian and Ferris (1967), during face-to-face conversations about feelings or attitudes, the actual words you say account for a mere 7% of your total communication, with voice tonality and body language making up the other 93%!

Whether you turn up for a meeting early, on time, late (or not at all) communicates something to the person waiting to meet with you—and you may not communicate what you intended due to their filters, including metaprograms being different from yours.

**Tip:** Decide on the image you would like to convey to your staff/patients/team, and make sure everything about you conveys that image—your attitude, your personal appearance, your communications with others (written and spoken), your behaviour and even your office/desk space!

## REFLECTION

- How does your 'behaviour' now support or undermine the image you would like to convey?

## *The Meaning of Your Communication Is the Response You Get*

While the words you use and your intention may be clear to you, it is the other person's interpretation and response that truly reflects the effectiveness of your communications. NLP teaches you the skills and flexibility to ensure that the message you send is the same as the message your patient/team receives.

Tip: If your communications are not generating the results you are hoping for, then ask a friend to listen to you, or read your written copy. You may find tweaking something very simple, such as changing key words or the underlying metaprogram, clarifies your messages and increases the positive responses you receive.

## REFLECTION

Think of a recent communication of yours which was not clear to others. How could that have been improved? What filter and/or metaprogram was contributing to any misunderstandings between you and who you were communicating with?

A challenge may be to explore how to effectively develop those NLP skills through creative learning opportunities such as coaching, peer mentoring, or action learning groups.

## Moving On to Creating Your Vision

So, now you are ready to create your vision. Being part of a 'vision' is a very empowering and motivating concept, and for it to motivate, everyone needs to be able identify with it. This is probably one of the most important aspects of personal development.

Without a vision, nobody actually knows where they are going or why. Look back at Dilts and DeLozier's model of logical levels: Vision or purpose sits at the top of this model, at the pinnacle of the triangle (or mountain!). A vision, whether it is a personal vision or the organisational vision, is what keeps everything else on track; it draws together every other level of the model.

Yet quite often, it is the one thing that is overlooked, as we become embroiled in day-to-day living, which mostly keeps us functioning at the environmental, behavioural and capability levels of the logical levels model. In health care, this often means ensuring that a caseload is managed and rosters are covered. While this is important, exceptional people and organisations move beyond this to having a clear overarching vision guiding the activities and roles for a common purpose.

Having a clear vision is what keeps us on track, helps us to achieve those goals, holds us to account and keeps us focussed when things get tough. Your personal vision serves as your reminder to yourself: Whom are you doing this for? Perhaps it is for your patients, your family, your children, your community, your country or to serve some higher religious calling?

Interestingly, monetary and material goals are not enough when it comes to creating a powerful vision. You need to identify why you are doing something as well as what you are hoping to achieve or gain for yourself.

Imagine we were standing by a 15-meter paddling pool and we said, 'We'll give you £10 to cross the paddling pool'. You would probably take your shoes off and paddle across straight away, just for the fun of it.

Now imagine we have swapped the paddling pool for a deep, fast-flowing river, about 15 meters across to the other bank. If we said, 'We'll give you £10 to swim across', would you do it? We suspect you would say 'no' straightaway because it's not worth it.

Now imagine the same scenario, only this time, your child or loved one is on the other side of the river, and they are in danger. How quickly would you be in the river and swimming to the other side as fast as you could, because the reason for doing it is now a lot more powerful?

For your vision to be powerful, it has to be something which ignites your passion, fires up your potential and motivates you so much that you will stick at it, however challenging life gets and regardless of how many obstacles get put in your way.

For your personal vision to be motivational and empowering, you need to take full ownership of it and make sure it is *your* vision for your life. When you have identified your personal vision, check that it really belongs to you, aligns with your values and comes from your heart, rather than being something you think others expect of you. In challenging times especially, you will find that your vision needs to be compelling, to fire you with passion and be able to motivate you into digging deep within yourself to take that next step.

A departmental or organisational vision has the same effect—it keeps individuals and teams on track, enables them to achieve their goals and keeps everyone focussed when the going gets tough! Obviously, any higher vision has not necessarily been created by each individual, and yet still needs to create motivation and passion in everyone, either because it complements personal visions or it resonates enough to inspire others individually or as part of a team. Communicating and selling the vision then is also vitally important to its success. (Chapters 5 and 6 explore leading others and teams and inspiring them to get on board with your vision.)

## Before Writing Your Vision, You Need to Recognise Your Power Base

One of the most important effects NLP can have on anyone is to empower them to the realisation that they are in control of their thoughts, their emotions and therefore their behaviour. In other words, *they* are their own power base.

Many NLP models have been successfully taught to adult care workers and parents over the last few years as part of a course called 'Managing High Functioning Autism, Aspergers and ADHD using NLP'. This was funded by Hertfordshire County Council in England because they recognised the positive impact of these courses on their adult services budget (Cunningham 2009).

The models that were taught had a great impact on the adult care workers because they were then better able to understand how the people in their care ended up exhibiting some of their negative behaviours.

Through this greater understanding, the care workers were able to intervene in different ways, showing behavioural flexibility and recognising the possible triggers for negative behaviour far earlier in the process. They were also able to empower the people in their care by teaching them some of the models, where relevant, on an individual basis to improve self-management abilities of the clients.

The course showed how adults can access and recognise their power base to make a difference.

## Having Recognised Your Power Base, You Need to Establish an Inner Confidence to Put It into Practice

Many things contribute towards establishing an inner confidence, including having congruence within yourself, as mentioned previously. If you can experience congruence across every one of Dilts and DeLozier's logical levels (i.e., that every level is supporting your inner drive and identity as a leader), then a level of inner confidence, self-awareness and groundedness will be established and maintained.

Of course, in many situations, gaining this congruence is the challenge! The first step is to have an awareness that incongruence between those levels is what is 'wobbling' the inner confidence. This awareness can be identified using a simple exercise.

## ACTIVITY

*Refer to the neurological levels diagram (Figure 2.1) in Chapter 2.*

Make some big labels representing the logical-levels environment—environment, behaviours, capabilities, beliefs and values, identity and vision (or purpose)— and lay these out on the floor in front of you, with environment nearest to you and vision furthest away, so you can take one step forward into each level.

Then identify your vision (or your team vision or company vision, if these are more appropriate) and step into the first section (environment). Whilst you are standing in this section, become curious and explore how environment may be affecting your vision, both positively or negatively, and check whether your environment is aligned with your vision, i.e., see if there is congruence in this section. You may find there is good alignment already, and you may find there are little (or big) tweaks to be made in order to bring your environment more in line with your vision, thus contributing to your inner confidence and peace of mind.

Continue to take steps up to each level, exploring and questioning each one as you go. You may find as you step up the levels, that something else comes to light, and this may impact on the other levels. If this is the case, then step back into the previous level and realign that one, based upon what you have discovered higher up.

The aim of this exercise is to evaluate your logical levels in a particular context and identify where any incongruence may lie. Use this to provide insights into the most effective way to create positive change.

The higher the logical level at which any intervention is made, potentially the more impact on the lower levels. For example, redecorating the ward office will only affect staff productivity if it was the environment which was affecting productivity in the first place. If staff members don't believe in themselves and their ability to do their job effectively, the money set aside for redecoration may be better invested in staff development, which would increase capabilities, improve staff morale and lead to increased productivity.

## ACTIVITY

So, now you understand yourself and have a good understanding of others. Are you ready to articulate your purpose or vision? What is it that gets you out of bed to go to work? On a good day, what was it that motivated you and left you feeling good about what you had done? Beyond managing your caseload, what is the purpose of your department and how do you align with that? How do you add value to it? Think of a day when you loved your work: What was it about that day that made the difference?

Take some time to reflect on what you do and what you would like to do in the future. As Stephen Covey (2006) said, 'What legacy do you want to leave?' What mark do you want to make? Using whatever words, artefacts or pictures that come to you, just sketch out your vision, your purpose, giving it life and energy so that you are genuinely excited about what you plan to do in the future. Being able to explain why that excites you—what will that give you? Find a form of words that encapsulates that so you can share it with someone else to bring your vision into being. Assume that anything is possible!

You have now set your future direction. You can go back and add in details, and you can work out the 'how' over time—but you have placed in your future path a bright positive picture of what you want. That's a huge step in your leadership journey. Take time to imagine how great you will feel when you achieve that, and of course you can come back time and time again to update and revise your vision.

## In Conclusion

As Riggio (2009) explained, great leaders are not always born that way and, unfortunately, many leadership training programs don't sufficiently emphasise the importance of understanding yourself. Becoming a successful leader is a journey towards our own self-development: It is more about the process than the end point. In order to lead others, we need to be able to relate to and connect with them, their motivations, their needs and aspirations, and their deepest values and core beliefs—and that takes ongoing commitment to achieve.

*Authentic leadership* is a term often referred to because, before others are willing to be led by us, they will want to connect to something within us—something that is authentic, real and true. They want to know what we stand for—our vision—before deciding whether or not to follow. Within this chapter, we have discussed ways to identify our vision, what is important to us and how to create a mind-set for success. In order to be authentic leaders, we need to be a person that others can relate to. We need to know ourselves, our beliefs and values, and how they manifest in our attitudes, behaviours and actions and in the impact that we have on others. Then we have to be willing to flex and adapt to achieve success.

Vision in leadership is very powerful. It draws commitment from people as they see and share our vision, feeling like they want to be part of it. Visionary leadership motivates the individual, team and organisation. Visionary leaders know where they want to get to because they have a sense of purpose and a clear guide as to how to get there. The vision will captivate people, driving their attention and focus while empowering their own sense of self and the role that they play within the team. A vision begins with a thought or an idea, but when put into action, it can change teams, communities and even nations! Where will your vision take you?

# References

Bandler, R., and J. Grinder. 1979. *Frogs into princes*. Moab, UT: Real People Press.

Charvet, S. R. 1997. *Words that change minds: Mastering the language of influence*. Dubuque, IA: Kendall/Hall.

Covey, S. 2006. *The 8th habit: From effectiveness to greatness*. New York: Simon & Schuster.

Cunningham, E. M. 2009. Hertfordshire County Council recognises the positive effects of NLP. *Rapport*, no. 15: 38–39. http://www.articlesbyevemenezescunningham.co.uk/sitebuildercontent/sitebuilderfiles/rapportnlpaspergers.pdf.

Dilts, R., and J. DeLozier. 2000. Perceptual positions. *Encyclopaedia of NLP*. NLP University Press. http://nlpuniversitypress.com/html2/PaPo30.html.

Ellerton, R. 2010. *Parents' handbook: NLP and common sense guide for family well-being*. Victoria, BC, Canada: Trafford Publishing.

Jung, C. G. 1971. *Psychological Types*, London: Routledge & Kegan Paul.

Mehrabian, Albert and Ferris, Susan R. 1967. Inference of attitudes from nonverbal communication in two channels. *Journal of Consulting Psychology*, vol. 31(3), Jun 1967, 248–252. doi: 10.1037/h0024648

Myers, I. 2000. *Introduction to Type* (6th ed.). Oxford, England: OPP Ltd.

Riggio, R. E. 2009. Leaders: Born or made? The most often-asked question about leadership, and the answer is: *Psychology Today* March 18. http://www.psychologytoday.com/blog/cutting-edge-leadership/200903/leaders-born-or-made.

# 4 Models of Communication Excellence

Suzanne Henwood and Lisa Booth

So, now you have a vision and you want to share it.

## Communication in Leadership

Communication is a core skill within leadership: It sits at the very core of influencing effectively. It is essential in building relationships and reaching goals. What may be less familiar is the concept that communication is not only with others, or externally focussed, but also with self. Internal communication—how we drive and lead ourselves and influence the decisions we make—is also an important skill which appears to be less frequently discussed. It is also fundamental in how we communicate with ourselves, as outlined in Chapter 2.

The heart of communication in leadership is around purposeful influence, being very aware of the impact of any communication (to self and others) and assessing whether or not it moves you towards your desired outcome, or whether indeed it inhibits and alienates in some way, albeit unintentionally. Effective leaders choose how they communicate, with a very deliberate focus and a desired outcome in mind.

In this chapter we will be focusing on two powerful communication models: NLP (Neuro-Linguistic Programming) and TA (Transactional Analysis). Within NLP, some of the processes within communication are beautifully explored, allowing you to understand why people communicate differently and why two people might physically hear the same message, yet create a very different interpretation of it, to which they then respond. In NLP the emphasis is on you holding the responsibility within any interaction, taking responsibility not only for the outgoing message, but also for the response you receive from another person and adjusting your communication if you do not get the response you want. In TA, we are offered a deep understanding of these levels of communication, which allows a different understanding of the interactions between people in practice.

While we cannot fully explore both models in depth in one chapter, what we aim to do is to introduce you to the two models and offer some approaches to exploring those models in practice and applying them to your context to enhance communication.

# Neuro-Linguistic Programming

NLP was developed in the 1970s and has a variety of definitions. There are a plethora of books and websites that can be accessed to find more detail. Some of our favourite resources related to the workplace are listed in Resource Box 4.1.

The NLP communication model

This simple, yet profound model demonstrates some key components of understanding the communication process (Figure 4.1):

1. Information from the outside world is perceived and taken internally through our five senses (as is information coming from our gut and/ or heart and brain, as discussed in mBraining.com (and introduced

## Box 4.1 Resource

*NLP and Coaching for Health Care Professionals: Developing Expert Practice*

Suzanne Henwood and Jim Lister (2007)

One of the few books written for healthcare practitioners in relation to clinical practice.

*NLP at Work*

Sue Knight offers an excellent introductory text to the full range of NLP tools and techniques for people at work (though not specifically about health care, the text can be easily applied by the reader to any work setting).

ANLP.org

This is an excellent website for accessing information and resources about NLP. ANLP is an independent body overseeing NLP practice, predominantly (but not exclusively) in the UK, and is a great place to start looking for NLP trainers or publications.

http://nlpuniversitypress.com/

An excellent encyclopaedia of NLP for those who want more depth about NLP processes and terminology.

**Communication Model**

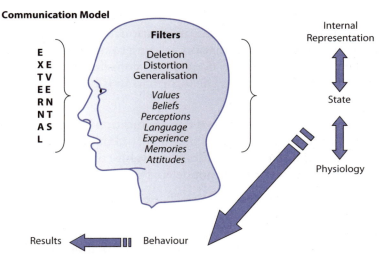

**Figure 4.1** NLP communication model (Henwood and Lister 2007)

in Chapter 16), so that, for example, emotions felt in the heart and sense of identity from the gut are also 'processed' in the head).

2. The information from all sources is passed through a range of filters to reduce the volume of data to manageable levels and to help us to make sense of what we are perceiving.

3. The filtered information leads to information being processed in one of three ways: deleted, distorted or generalised (see below for more details).

4. An internal representation of the external information is then brought to our consciousness: a representation of 'reality' which is unique to the individual (often called our 'map' — this is our version of reality, not the reality itself).

5. That internal representation generates an emotional response: 'our state'.

6. This in turn determines our physiology—or our physical reaction seen externally.

7. The combination of Internal Representation + State + Physiology determines our behaviour.

8. Our behaviours determine our results.

For example, information can be

**Deleted:** The process by which some information is taken note of, while other bits of information are 'overlooked'.

For example, you, as a clinical leader, are concerned with waiting times, and you are chasing staff to complete a set of audit sheets that you have left out for them in the department. Yet, for the second month running, staff are not complying. It may be that, due to an internal filter, those staff are not placing any importance on that information. So they hear you on some level, and then delete that information, leading to no responses within the audit data set. It may be they do not even consciously hear you discuss the audit in the staff meeting, as the information is deleted at a very early stage.

In order to increase the chance of that communication being heard and to improve the chances of it being acted on, you could think about relaying the information to staff differently, building on a value you know is of importance to them so that the information is not deleted prior to it being acted on.

Use your knowledge of metaprograms (Chapter 3) to appeal to both towards and away-from motivation, verbally 'mark' or 'emphasise' a point through tone, repetition or saying 'this is important because...'. Ensure you plan what to say to avoid overload or unnecessary detail that detracts from your key message. And remember to appeal to staff values (what is important to them), weaving that into your communication whilst also explaining why it is important to you and your values, and how it contributes to the wider vision.

Understanding that information is deleted is important. It is not deliberate, and is not always conscious, and we all do it.

## REFLECTION

What information can you think of that has been deleted by staff, or by patients, or by yourself? Reflecting on that now, what could you have done differently to have ensured that the communication was not filtered out?

**Distorted:** Distortion is where we in some way change what we are perceiving to create a new 'truth'.

Information can be distorted when you hear a message coming in, or you take in visual information. Having compared it to previously stored information, you then distort what you have really seen to make it fit what you have stored inside, or what you thought you would see or wanted to see. An example of this is seeing someone you think you recognise, but when you approach the person you realise it is not the person you thought it was.

In clinical practice, this can be apparent, for example, when reading a set of X-rays or patient notes, or reviewing a patient history, with a predetermined idea of the pathology you will find, because of known history, or previous examples you have successfully treated. A lady who has just given birth, for example, feeling unwell, may have a systemic infection missed because you focus on maternity-related issues and you expect the lady at that stage not to feel 100%.

In a more positive way, distortion can be used creatively to visualise what something might be if it were done differently, how a new room might look with new equipment, how a new protocol would operate in practice following successful introduction.

**Generalised:** Where different experiences are compared and where conclusions are reached that may not be completely accurate.

Just being aware of this can help to avoid unresourceful distortions in practice.

For example, you have to obtain consent from a child of 12 years of age. You may have previously encountered this twice and found that each time the child was unable to understand sufficiently to give consent, so parents were brought in. There is a risk that you then determine all children of that age are unable to give consent, which may not be the case in reality.

Generalisations can also be positive, leading to fast learning. For example, a nurse can probably transfer knowledge and experience about dressings and does not have to relearn how to use each new style of dressing introduced.

Being able to recognise that these three processes are in active operation (in yourself and others), and being able to ask specific questions to recapture some of the lost detail, can be empowering.

Examples of working with those processes in practice:

Statement:

*She never lets me have any time off for development—she hates me.*

Deletion: Who?

Distortion: How does her denying you time off for development mean she hates you?

Generalisation: 'Never' can be easily broken down by asking 'what never?'

Statement:

*I didn't get the job—they are never going to promote me here.*

Deletion: Who exactly?

Distortion: How do know you will never get a promotion here?

Generalisation: Can you think of anyone else who was unsuccessful at first attempt and got a promotion later?

What is deleted, distorted and generalised is determined by our filters. We listed a few common filters in the diagram of the NLP communication model, above, and values have already been explored in Chapter 3. Take time to reflect on your own filters and how they are affecting your communication in practice.

## REFLECTION

Using the examples we have listed, can you identify some of your filters which may impact on your behaviours? For example:

*Values*: What is important to you about your profession? Or about leadership?

*Beliefs*: What do you believe about patient-centred care or leadership style?

*Language*: How might language or medical terminology or professional acronyms act as filters?

*Experience*: How might previous experience filter information in your patients' map of reality?

*Attitudes*: How might your attitudes towards something or someone change how you see reality?

Asking specific questions (of others and yourself) can help to recover some of the deletions, distortions and generalisations and will uncover individual interpretations that have been made as to what has been experienced. Challenging internal representations that we took as 'true' and uncovering misunderstandings that may be impacting on professional relationships can be very powerful. Now that you know about these filters, you will find you can reflect more deeply on communication effectiveness.

## Working above the Line

In Chapter 3 we introduced the NLP concept of being 'at cause' or 'at effect'. When we are 'at cause', we take responsibility for ourselves and our behaviours. The NLP communication model really assists us in doing that. When we are 'at effect', we are happy to maintain distortions so that we can blame others for the results we are achieving. Leaders are people who spend most of their time 'at cause'. They take responsibility for the outcomes and change their behaviours if they are not getting the results they desire.

In health care this is also a great model for understanding patients' behaviours. For example, have you ever been on call when a patient gets aggressive, impatient or abusive? This model enables you to think through what their internal representation might be and what alternative interpretation might be possible. For example, take time:

To explain any delays, to avoid distortions which might have a less than positive meaning (they don't care, they are not taking me seriously, they are lazy).

To look up any previous history, for example, the last time a patient had to have three bloods taken, so that you can understand and manage any potential anxiety appropriately, rather than seeing the patient as being 'difficult'.

To handle complaints by asking the patients what they want and what is important to them, thereby immediately ensuring you relate to their filters (values, perceptions, experience, etc.) and acknowledge their 'reality', rather than assuming you know what the issues are, thus saving time and reducing patient frustration.

This brief look at the NLP communication model shows how it can raise self-awareness, increase our understanding of self and others and enhance our flexibility as to how we respond in any situation. By exploring how we impact on the 'internal representation' of any reality, thereby creating our state (or how we feel about any situation), we can really begin to see how we have much more control of our behaviours in practice, which is a key to great leadership—managing self in practice. We believe the NLP communication model is a powerful model for transforming communication in a healthcare environment and would urge all practitioners to become familiar with it. It will be invaluable to you as a leader as you coach and mentor others through difficult situations by offering a whole new level of reflection.

# Transactional Analysis

Transactional Analysis (TA), developed by the psychiatrist Eric Berne in the 1960s, is a tool that can be used by anyone to analyse interactions between individuals. The goal is to identify our interaction styles and 'choose' how to improve our relationships. Like NLP's theory around 'at cause', TA theory believes that we are responsible for the outcomes of communication and that we can change our behaviour if we are not achieving the desired effect. The basic components of TA are: ego-states, egograms, transactions, life scripts and games. More detail on these can be found using the resources outlined in Resource Box 4.2.

## Box 4.2 Resource

*I'm OK, You're OK*
Tom Harris (1969), New York: HarperCollins
A very good book that outlines why we behave as we do according to our life scripts.

*Working It Out at Work: Understanding Attitudes and Building Relationships*
Julie Hay (2009), Watford, UK: Sherwood Publishing

*TA: 100 Key Points and Techniques*
Mark Widdowson (2009), Routledge
An introductory text to the concepts of TA and the underlying theory. Some very good practical examples given.

TAstudent.org.uk
A good website for accessing information and further resources about TA.

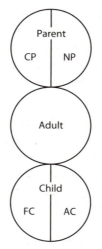

**Figure 4.2** A PAC diagram demonstrating the three ego-states and their subdivisions

## Ego-States

According to Berne (1998), our personality is made up of three basic components: the Parent, the Adult and the Child (see Figure 4.2). These ego-states are in place by the time we are 5 years old and are the feelings/memories associated with communication events when we were younger. When we face a similar communication event in later life, these feelings are recalled, and we react in ways that are reminiscent of those earlier communication events (Hollins 2011).

According to Hollins (2011), the Parent is subdivided into the Controlling Parent (CP) and the Nurturing Parent (NP). The Controlling Parent criticises, finds fault and is judgemental of others. It uses words such as *no, can't, shouldn't*; the Nurturing Parent, by contrast, offers advice, is sympathetic and caring. The Adult is the logical and rational part of our personality; it makes decisions in the 'here and now', asks questions and is analytical. The Child, like the Parent, is subdivided into the Free Child (FC) and the Adapted Child (AC). The Free Child is fun, spontaneous, breaks the rules and is essentially uninhibited. Conversely, the Adapted Child conforms, uses words such as *sorry, please, thank you*. It learns the accepted behaviours of a culture; however, if the Adapted Child receives too many Critical Parent responses, it can become submissive.

## REFLECTION

- How many of those states do you recognise in yourself?
- Which do you operate from mostly when you lead?

# Egograms

Although we are all capable of expressing ourselves from any one of these ego-states, what makes us unique is how these ego-states dominate in our personality. We can assess how dominant these ego-states might be using the egogram checklist developed by Ishikawa and Iwai in 1975 (cited in Shirai 2006). According to Ishikawa and Iwai, an egogram is a psychological fingerprint, with each person having a unique profile that can be seen and measured.

Complete the egogram checklist in Table 4.1. Using the following four options:

(0) Seldom

(1) Sometimes

(2) Often

(3) Always

Put your answer on the white square in columns 1–5 of each question. Don't think too hard about each question; put down the first answer that comes into your head.

**Table 4.1:** Egogram Checklist

| | | Column number | | | | |
|---|---|:---:|:---:|:---:|:---:|:---:|
| | | 1 | 2 | 3 | 4 | 5 |
| 1 | You behave efficiently and briskly | □ | ■ | □ | ■ | □ |
| 2 | You are an open-minded and free person | □ | ■ | ■ | □ | ■ |
| 3 | You look down on others | ■ | □ | ■ | □ | □ |
| 4 | You can adjust yourself well to others | □ | ■ | ■ | ■ | □ |
| 5 | You respect traditions | ■ | □ | ■ | ■ | ■ |
| 6 | You recognise others strengths and praise them | □ | ■ | ■ | ■ | ■ |
| 7 | You express your sympathy with others well | □ | □ | ■ | ■ | ■ |
| 8 | You make a decision observing reality well | □ | ■ | □ | ■ | ■ |
| 9 | You show your feelings quickly on your face | □ | ■ | ■ | □ | ■ |
| 10 | You are critical of things | ■ | □ | ■ | □ | ■ |
| 11 | You are a reserved and passive person | ■ | ■ | ■ | ■ | □ |
| 12 | You are very thoughtful of others | □ | ■ | ■ | □ | ■ |
| 13 | You put off things you don't like by using excuses | □ | ■ | □ | ■ | ■ |
| 14 | You cherish a sense of responsibility | ■ | □ | ■ | □ | ■ |

continued …

Models of Communication Excellence

| 15 | You talk to others face to face with a straight back |
| 16 | You have many complaints and dissatisfactions |
| 17 | You take care of other people well |
| 18 | You look into other people's facial expressions |
| 19 | You respond to others saying why/how? |
| 20 | You are moralistic |
| 21 | You judge things accurately |
| 22 | You express your surprise with oh! and/or wow! |
| 23 | You are strict to other's failures and weaknesses |
| 24 | You cook, wash and clean enthusiastically |
| 25 | You hesitate to speak out what you are thinking |
| 26 | You are good at making excuses |
| 27 | You often say to others 'you should…' |
| 28 | You don't like to sit still or be inactive |
| 29 | You obey rules and regulations strictly |
| 30 | You relate yourself to others well |
| 31 | You try to please other people |
| 32 | You can say what you want to say without hesitating |
| 33 | You gather all kinds of information and think |
| 34 | You are self-centred |
| 35 | You often say 'excuse me' and or 'I'm sorry' |
| 36 | You make a decision without mixing up your feelings |
| 37 | You have a strong sense of curiosity |
| 38 | You don't pay too much attention to what others think |
| 39 | You pursue your ideals |
| 40 | You make plans carefully before you carry them out |
| 41 | You do not become emotional when you talk |
| 42 | You console people who are in trouble |
| 43 | You take the initiative in volunteer activities |
| 44 | You express your opinions clearly and firmly |
| 45 | You make a decision on intuition, not with reason |
| 46 | You are flexible |
| 47 | You want to obtain what you want persistently |
| 48 | You can forgive others for their mistakes generously |
| 49 | You can talk to other people freely |
| 50 | You cannot say 'no' to others when asked to do things |

Now add up the scores for each column and record them in Table 4.2.

**Table 4.2:** Score

| Score | Column 1 | Column 2 | Column 3 | Column 4 | Column 5 |
|---|---|---|---|---|---|
| 32 | | | | | |
| 30 | | | | | |
| 28 | | | | | |
| 26 | | | | | |
| 24 | | | | | |
| 22 | | | | | |
| 20 | | | | | |
| 18 | | | | | |
| 16 | | | | | |
| 14 | | | | | |
| 12 | | | | | |
| 10 | | | | | |
| 8 | | | | | |
| 6 | | | | | |
| 4 | | | | | |
| 2 | | | | | |
| Score | CP (Controlling Parent) | NP (Nurturing Parent) | A (Adult) | FC (Free Child) | AC (Adapted Child) |

**Table 4.3:** The Transactional Analysis Subscales of the Adjective Checklist (ACL)

| Controlling Parent (CP) | Nurturing Parent (NP) | Adult (A) | Free Child (FC) | Adapted Child (AC) |
|---|---|---|---|---|
| Autocratic | Affectionate | Alert | Adventurous | Anxious |
| Bossy | Considerate | Capable | Affectionate | Apathetic |
| Demanding | Forgiving | Clear thinking | Artistic | Argumentative |
| Dominant | Generous | Efficient | Energetic | Arrogant |
| Fault finding | Gentle | Fair minded | Enthusiastic | Awkward |
| Forceful | Helpful | Logical | Excitable | Complaining |
| Intolerant | Kind | Methodical | Humorous | Confused |
| Nagging | Praising | Organised | Imaginative | Defensive |
| Opinionated | Sympathetic | Precise | Natural | Dependent |
| Prejudiced | Tolerant | Rational | Pleasure seeking | Hurried |
| Rigid | Understanding | Realistic | Sexy | Inhibited |
| Severe | Unselfish | Reasonable | Spontaneous | Moody |
| Stern | Warm | Unemotional | Uninhibited | Nervous |

*Source:* Williams and Williams (1980)

What you have drawn here is an egogram of your own personality. For a fuller understanding of the sorts of behaviours you will be displaying when you are interacting in one of those ego-states, see the TA subscales (Table 4.3) of the Adjective Checklist (ACL). The ACL is also an important tool in helping us understand others as it allows us to identify other people's ego-states. The adjectives tell us that it is important to listen to 'how' something is being said, not 'what' is being said, i.e., active listening. Look out for non-verbal clues such as a lack of eye contact, slumped posture, tone of voice, etc.

It is important to know your dominant ego-state, as this will certainly influence your communication and leadership style (Weihrich 1979), as you have the greatest dependence on that ego-state (Hollins 2011). According to Dusay, when we are in stressful situations, the ego-state which scored highest on the checklist will dominate more than when we are not stressed (cited in Shirai 2006).

## REFLECTION

- What is your dominant ego-state? How might this affect your behaviour under stress?

- Now that you know your dominant ego-state, how might this affect your interactions with others?

## Complementary and Crossed Transactions

Quite simply, we communicate from an ego-state and aim it at another ego-state. If we get a response from where we aimed the stimulus, then this will be a complementary transaction. As we all want to be in a complementary transaction, knowing how to achieve them can be an important step in building rapport with others. The most common and

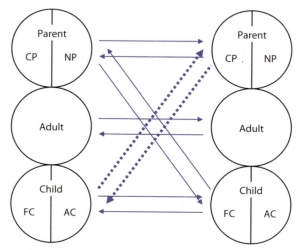

**Figure 4.3** The most common complementary transactions

naturally occurring complementary transactions are demonstrated in Figure 4.3. For further information on complementary transactions, read Widdowson (2009).

For example, imagine a colleague is complaining, anxious and upset because he or she cannot cope with their workload; according to the ACL (Table 4.3), this individual is in the Adapted Child ego-state. Where are you most likely to respond from? It is likely that your natural instinct will be to exhibit affection, sympathy, find out what is wrong and offer support and advice (Stewart and Joines 1987). According to the ACL (Table 4.3), this is your Nurturing Parent ego-state responding to an Adapted Child stimulus. This type of interaction is demonstrated using the dashed-arrow effect in Figure 4.3.

When we are in a complementary transaction, the communication runs smoothly. After all, both parties are getting the responses that they want. Therefore, we want to be in a complementary transaction, but this does not mean that all complementary transactions are positive. Think back to the example of the colleague who is upset (AC). By stimulating a response from your NP, the colleague receives help and support, and in some cases you may even end up doing some of the work for the individual. This colleague then learns that to get the desired help, all that he or she needs to do is display AC behaviours and you will provide that help, i.e., an unproductive cycle begins. This is an area of TA known as 'game playing'. The term *game* should not suggest that these are fun to play. The aim of the game is to make another person feel bad (see Figure 4.4). The characteristic of a game is that the communication has a social level, i.e., what is said, and a psychological undertone. For this reason, they are known as ulterior transactions, i.e., they have an ulterior motive. It is also worth noting that games are played from complementary ego-states. Again, Tom Harris (1969) gives a very good explanation of games and is worth reading if you want to know more about this area of TA.

This is where another facet of TA can come in useful. Crossed transactions are when a stimulus does not get an expected response (Figure 4.5). Just as complementary transactions can be positive or negative, so can crossed transactions. If a crossed transaction is used to break an unproductive cycle of communication, then this would be a positive use of crossing a transaction, e.g., the colleague who is struggling with the workload (AC) may rethink her strategy if the responses she receives are Adult in nature.

| I'm OK | I'm Not OK |
|---|---|
| You're OK | You're OK |
| I'm OK | I'm Not OK |
| You're Not OK | You're Not OK |

**Figure 4.4** The OK corral

*Stimulus*: 'I just can't manage; I don't know what to do about all this work' (AC).

*Response*: 'Try prioritising what is most important. Write out a list and see if that helps you identify the urgent work' (A).

Remember, we want to be in a complementary transaction; we want communication to run smoothly and to get a good outcome for both parties. Therefore, when we find ourselves in a crossed transaction, we 'shift' to complement the other person's stimulus. By crossing the transaction with the Adult ego-state, we encourage the other person to do the same.

However, if we cross transactions in an attempt to dismiss, put down or control another person, then this would be a negative use of these interactions, for example:

*Stimulus*: 'I just can't manage; I don't know what to do about all this work' (AC wanting an NP response).

*Response*: 'I've got enough of my own work to do without doing yours for you as well' (CP).

Although the response is still from the Parent ego-state, the fact that the person struggling with the workload wanted a Nurturing Parent response means that she did not get the response she wanted (see Figure 4.5). Therefore, a negative crossed transaction has occurred, and as Hollins (2011) points out, if the AC gets too much CP attention, this can result in anxious, defensive and submissive behaviours.

To establish whether we are in a complementary or crossed transaction and how we might make communication more productive, we need to ask ourselves certain questions in a certain order and note them on a

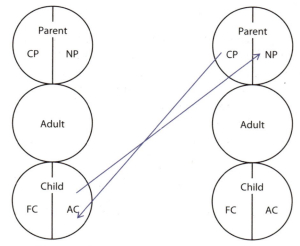

**Figure 4.5** A crossed transaction

PAC diagram. It is certainly worth doing this if you feel that you are in an interaction that doesn't seem to be achieving your objectives.

## REFLECTION

Think of a recent difficult communication event and ask yourself:

1. What ego-state am I interacting from? (Be honest here, and use the ACL (Table 4.3) to diagnose your ego-state.)

2. To which ego-state am I aiming this stimulus? (Think about the response you want by looking at the behaviours on the ACL [Table 4.3] and the natural complementary transactions that exist [Figure 4.3].) Draw a line on your PAC diagram to indicate which ego-state you are communicating from to the ego-state you want to respond.

3. From which ego-state do I get a response? (Again, use the ACL to diagnose the other person's ego-state.) Draw a second line on your PAC diagram from the ego-state that responds, to the initial ego-state you communicated with.

4. Is the transaction crossed or complementary?

5. Am I using the best ego-state to stimulate the response that I want? For example, if you want an Adult response, then you need to use your Adult ego-state to elicit this. If you want a Child response, then you need to be using your Parent or Child (depending on the situation). Think about the interactions that naturally occur (see Figure 4.3). It never ceases to amaze me when individuals want an Adult ego-state response, but think they will get this using a CP stimulus.

## REFLECTION

Using both models, think of a critical incident that did not go as well as you would have liked. What might have been happening to prevent a great outcome, and what can you do differently in the future to enhance the outcome further for all parties, using these two models?

# Summary

In both NLP and TA, it is clear that increased understanding and awareness gives you an opportunity to more purposefully direct your communication. When done with respect and a genuine valuing and concern for others, this can be incredibly powerful and lead to significantly enhanced performance.

We recommend you add these two tools to your leader's toolbox and take time out to reflect on critical incidents involving communication issues, maybe a conflict or misunderstanding as well as an interaction that went really well, and use the tools to give insight into how you could have got even better results.

# References

Berne, E. 1998. *What do you say after you say hello?* 19th ed., Corgi edition. London: Transworld.

Bolden, K. 1996a. Transactional analysis: Part 1. *Practise Nursing* 7 (12): 24–28.

Bolden, K. 1996b. Transactional analysis: Part 2. *Practise Nursing* 7 (13): 40–42.

Harris, T. 1969. *I'm OK, you're OK*. New York: HarperCollins.

Hay, J. 2009. *Working it out at work: Understanding attitudes and building relationships*. Watford, UK: Sherwood.

Henwood, S. M., and J. Lister. 2007. *NLP and coaching for healthcare professionals: Developing expert practise*. Chichester, UK: John Wiley and Sons.

Hollins, C. 2011. Transactional analysis: A method of analysing communication. *British Journal of Midwifery* 19 (9): 587–93.

Shirai, S. 2006. How transactional analysis can be used in terminal care. *International Congress Series* 1287: 179–84.

Stewart, I., and V. Joines. 1987. *Transactional analysis today: A new introduction to transactional analysis*. Chapel Hill, NC: Lifespace Publishing.

Weihrich, H. 1979. How to change a leadership pattern. *Management Review* 68 (4): 26–40.

Widdowson, M. 2009. *TA: 100 key points and techniques*. London: Routledge.

Williams, K., and J. Williams. 1980. The assessment of transactional analysis ego-states via the adjective checklist. *Journal of Personality Assessment* 44 (2): 120–28.

# 5 The Art of Followership

David Collier and Jennifer Haven

When recruiters appoint a leader, they often ask questions about the business, strategic direction and leadership expertise. A person with reasonable experience can provide answers which place them in the best profile for this role. Yet they seldom ask the key question 'Who (and how) will you be leading?' The question is not the same as 'What sort of leader are you?' This chapter explores concepts of followership, recognising that leading others is in fact the art of cultivating followers: a dance, constantly changing and evolving as you as leader and your followers grow and adapt to changing contexts. The focus on followership reflects a move from traditional leadership structures based around power, expertise and recognition, to those which rely on collaboration, personal responsibility and service delivery without compromising the leader's function. In understanding this, the reasons why leaders need followers become even more apparent.

## Followership

The Kings Fund in the UK commissioned a report on followership in the National Health Service. The report said that 'followership is the anvil of leadership—the former can make or break the latter' (Grint and Holt 2011). The statement reflects recognition of the power of followers. Followers have the skills, knowledge and opportunity to create upward influence within an organisation (Daft and Pirola-Merlo 2009), yet further than this, they hold a key role in attaining success. The concept is well demonstrated in an entertaining and popular video entitled 'How to Start a Movement' (Sivers 2010). The video shows a person dancing unconventionally whilst others sit and observe. The first follower then boldly joins the leader, and he is welcomed as an equal (Sivers 2010). Together they proceed to invite others to join them. As momentum builds, people become engaged, the leader gains followers and a movement ensues. The lesson is simple; without followers, the leader stands alone.

Philosophically, the art of followership goes to the crux of who a person is, their personality, the personal leadership concepts they follow and the manner and values they bring to others. Anyone who has worked in a large organisation will have encountered all styles of leadership, perhaps in equal measure. Your responses to the leaders you have met and worked with have shaped your ideas about leadership. You are encouraged to reflect on these experiences, consider the types of leaders that you have followed and what it was about that leader that encouraged you to engage with them.

## REFLECTION

Whom do you choose to follow and why?

Climbing mountains is a great metaphor for allowing us to better understand the relationships in following and leadership. When the team identifies the mountain that they are planning to climb together, they are, in an organisational sense, setting the vision. It follows from this that the mission statement which accompanies the vision is simply, in climbing terms, the question as to why we are climbing this mountain as distinct from any other. Again, it follows logically that we should also have a philosophy underpinning our journey, namely how we will treat each other as we travel: our values. If we return to the healthcare context, followers may initially come together through a common desire to work within the hospital environment, with a vision to help people, a common goal to improve health outcomes and core values that make a positive difference to peoples' lives. Sharing this vision and philosophy can engage those with similar views and thus cultivate followers. However, this is not the case for all healthcare practitioners, with some joining the professions for status, power, familiarity or sometimes convenience. The question then is how to engage all followers as a cohesive team that is capable of 'climbing mountains' and overcoming challenges together as one unit.

Lovegrove and Long (2012, 230), in the context of the medical imaging profession, said that 'effective responsible clinical leaders need equally effective responsible clinical followers'. If we reflect on the sort of leader that we wish to be, the answer is one that brings followers together as an effective team and empowers those followers to have ownership of their work and their workplace and to have responsibility for themselves. A leader's role is to develop followers into independent, critical thinkers and thus aid them in developing their own effectiveness (Daft and Pirola-Merlo 2009).

Effective followers hold a sense of responsibility and ownership for their own behaviour, for the consequences of their actions and for their own personal development (Daft and Pirola-Merlo 2009). Effective followers are active and able to demonstrate critical thinking, and they will challenge the leader to the point where they may even withdraw their support if they consider it necessary (Daft and Pirola-Merlo 2009). It is highly likely that you can identify those individuals within your own team, and yet equally possible that you are able to identify those who lack these qualities. Some followers are unable or unwilling to think critically in relation to the task at hand; they are referred to as *passive followers*, who will not challenge the status quo (Daft and Pirola-Merlo 2009). You may also be able to identify those who respond with cynicism or scepticism in relation to new endeavours. These individuals are described as *alienated followers*, who hold the ability to think critically, yet lack pro-active participation in problem-solving exercises. Whilst often highly capable, such persons may have had their enthusiasm marred by obstructive or oppressive leadership in the past (Daft and Pirola-Merlo 2009). In his seminal works on followership, Kelley (1992) presents a useful tool to identify these different followership styles in relation to one another.

Effective followers are key to developing the sense of collaboration and teamwork described in Chapter 6. Teams are supposed to run smoothly and concordantly; however, this is inherently challenging because of the differences that are evident in people, their personalities and their styles. As a result, there is a potential for disagreements, dysfunction and even disconnection in any group of followers. Whilst disconnection may be reflective of poor leadership, we must be careful to distinguish between the team which is comprehensively disconnected, those individuals who disconnect so as to avoid responsibility for themselves and those who choose not to follow because they do not believe in where they are to be led.

## When Followers Are Dysfunctional

Lencioni (2002) writes about five possible dysfunctions within a group of followers that originate from individual perceptions and personalities. The five dysfunctions are a lack of trust, a fear of conflict, a lack of commitment, an avoidance or lack of accountability and lack of attention to results.

There are two aspects to trust:

*Credibility*: The confidence that people will meet their end of a bargain, based on past experience.

*Exposure of vulnerability*: The trust that exposure of a person's weaknesses will not be used against him/her or the fact that statements made will not be used to victimise him/her.

Lencioni (2002) argues that *lack of trust* makes people fail to admit their weaknesses and shortfalls and, thus, fail to seek help. Lack of trust may also increase politicking and gossip. As a result, people may harbour grudges and be reluctant to offer their constructive feedback.

The second dysfunction identified by Lencioni (2002) is the *fear of conflict*. In many cases, it can be argued that followers have a fear of conflict because they also have a lack of trust. The inevitable consequence is that if followers avoid conflict, then the team can never engage in constructive debate. For some reason, and there are papers tackling this, the health professions are ones in which people avoid conflict because it so often is reported as potential victimisation. Leaders need their followers to engage in constructive conflict, and the leader's task is to have an environment in which such conflict is seen as fun, enjoyable and part of the environment. Strategically intelligent leadership will bring critical issues out for discussion amongst followers, ensuring that such conversations take place without the intrusion of personality or personal attacks. The leader's role in this is to guide the discussion and explore the ideas brought forward by the followers. The discussion must remain idea focussed so as to avoid political point scoring, one-upmanship or gossip. This takes time, but it is time well spent and worthy of encouraging and supporting, if only for the recognition of personal value that it brings to every individual.

The third dysfunction according to Lencioni (2002) is the *lack of commitment*. In managing upwards to boards of directors, healthcare leaders will all be aware that the board may have an agenda that they have not shared with management. The lack of candour inevitably results in a lack of commitment and, then, a failure to achieve the objectives desired by the governing body, all as a consequence of the lack of candid and open debate which can so easily eliminate fear of conflict. If leaders are to build followers with commitment, then the leaders must encourage their followers to construct unequivocal decisions that can be brought in, even without a complete consensus, and so allow the team to move on. When such commitment is hampered by a lack of certainty and consensus, this creates a dysfunction which slows decisions and paralyses activities of the group, creating distrust and lack of confidence.

Lencioni's (2002) fourth dysfunction is the *absence of accountability*. When followers remain unaccountable, this places undue pressure on others, including the leader. This attitude is frequently behind the comment, 'If I want the job done, I have to do it myself'. This leads to resentment within the team towards those individuals whose performance may not be equal to the rest. It also seems to increase mediocrity, as those who are not accountable may lose their pride and commitment to their work. All too frequently, the followers take refuge in a bureaucratic vision of what they are doing, which explains and justifies to them their frustration. The lack of accountability tends to vanish when the leaders clearly communicate the objectives and goals of the organisation so that everyone is sure of what is expected of them. Regular reviews and rewarding staff for good performance outside the review expectations are powerful tools in bringing about improved accountability. If rewards are used, they should also be distributed (if possible) so as to give the team a sense of collective responsibility.

The last of Lencioni's (2002) dysfunction points is that of *not focusing on results*. He argues that teams that pay attention to results tend to attain their goals because they have a focus point. Healthcare practitioners are expected to strive for evidence-based practice in their profession, and therefore a focus on results is not at odds with current thinking. Lencioni (2002) argues that within a group, individuals should constantly remind each other about their focus towards such achievements.

## REFLECTION

Which of these five dysfunctions do you recognise from teams you have worked in or with?

# Building Authentic Followers

The question for leaders, then, is to how to build genuine and robust trust amongst followers to promote effective collaboration. In this regard, the Johari Window is a valuable tool that can be used with simple training. Created by Joseph Luft and Harrington Ingham in 1955 in the United States, this tool empowers followers with sufficient understanding to admit weaknesses and mistakes and, thus, to ask for help in order to move forward (Luft 1984). They are able to accept other people's input without open indiscriminate critique in order to encourage their open participation. When performing the exercise, subjects are given a list of 56 adjectives, such as *calm*, *able*, *quiet*, *happy*, and are asked to select five or six that they feel describe their own personality. Peers of the subject are then given the same list, and each picks five or six adjectives that describe the subject. These adjectives are then mapped onto a grid.

Charles Handy (2000) calls this concept the Johari House with four rooms. Room 1 is the part of ourselves that we see and others see. Room 2 is the aspects that others see but we are not aware of. Room 3 is the most mysterious room, in that the unconscious or subconscious part of us is seen by neither ourselves nor others. Room 4 is our private space, which we know but keep from others. The concept is clearly related to the ideas propounded in the Myers-Briggs Type Indicator programme, which in turn derives from theories about the personality first explored by psychologist Carl Jung.

## REFLECTION

How do you communicate with followers?

When reflecting on followership styles and personality types it becomes obvious that there is no one-size-fits-all approach to engaging followers. Some may display a preference for face-to-face discussions and team meetings. Yet in the modern healthcare setting, it is not unusual for followers and leaders to connect through electronic platforms, including e-mail and social media. The latter approach has the capacity to overcome physical and logistical barriers to engagement and provides numerous advantages to both leaders and followers. Electronic platforms allow leaders to make philosophies, objectives and priorities explicit to all followers simultaneously. Leaders are also able to take note of followers' ideas and perspectives, a practice advocated by the Kings Fund (2011). For followers, the use of electronic media provides an opportunity to express themselves openly, without the limitation of their own personal inhibitions, inherently affecting face-to-face discussions. Followers can demonstrate initiative within the platform, thereby demonstrating their capacity as an effective follower. Further to this, they can emerge as an effective leader in their own right, holding the power to independently search for like-minded individuals, engage in conversation, generate and share knowledge, innovate, teach and learn (Kaplan and Haenlin 2010). Whilst several advantages have been made explicit, leaders must remain mindful of the challenges and potential risks of social media including abuse and misuse as well as intentional or inadvertent breaches of confidentiality. When reflecting on these key points, it is important to remember that followers are able to connect irrespective of whether the leader chooses to engage with the platform.

## REFLECTION

Consider your own personal and professional social media interactions:

- What do you gain from these interactions?
- What are the potential risks?

# How Social Media Is Impacting on Followership

Followers are able to fulfil a variety of needs through social media, above and beyond the obvious benefits of connection and communication (Shao 2009). Individuals are afforded emotional gratification, which may be centred on self or peer affirmation. They can also experience a range of emotions and feelings that they perceive to be unattainable in their own environment, including, for example, humour or empathy and pride or competence (Bartsch et al. 2006). Goleman (2006, p. 231), a seminal author of emotional and social intelligence theory, reminds us that our 'sense of our social value and status—and so our very self worth—comes from the cumulative messages we get from others about how they perceive us'. However, as likely as they are to experience positive connections, both leaders and followers are at risk of experiencing anxiety, fear and feelings of incompetence as they compare themselves to others within a social network (Bartsch et al. 2006). Thought must be given as to how staff can be affirmed and encouraged in their roles.

Leaders should be aware of the skills, experience and confidence that individual followers bring to the virtual environment. Miller (2011) highlights that individuals from Generation X grew up in the Internet era and are generally considered to be conversant with technologies and social media. The McCrindle Research (2013) report in Australia demonstrated little variation in Internet usage from individuals of Generation X, Generation Y and the Baby Boomers, yet the study also served as a reminder that there may be a difference in the choice of devices used to access the online world. Failure to appreciate the issues of accessibility—and comfort across all users—risks the introduction of a barrier to engagement.

Kaplan and Haenlin (2010) outline clear lessons for healthcare leaders considering social media interactions for cultivating or connecting with followers. Firstly: 'Be active, be interesting, be humble, be honest' (2010, pp. 66–67). They advocate a natural approach and the use of content that blends in with material posted by users. Having attempted such techniques in medical-imaging education, we can state that there is a definite balance between immersing yourself into the language and culture of the group whilst still modelling the appropriate communication that is expected of a health professional and leader in the field. In terms of selecting the appropriate media, Kaplan and Haelin (2010, pp. 66–67) advocate that leaders should 'choose carefully', make the application their own, align the online activity between different groups, ensure consistency of message across all channels and, most importantly, ensure access for all.

In the simplest of terms, then, leaders need followers so that they can be good leaders. Good leadership is characterised by humility on the part of a leader as to his or her role in creating the team and an intense pride on the part of the followers in being part of that leader's team. The open and supportive communication shared by all followers—as well as the clear recognition as to who is doing what, when and how—creates one of those teams which leaves those outside wondering how it came about.

# References

Bartsch, A., R. Mangold, R. Viehoff, and P. Vorderer. 2006. Emotional gratifications during media use: An integrative approach. *Communications* 31 (3): 261–78.

Daft, R. L., and A. Pirola-Merlo. 2009. *The leadership experience*. Melbourne, Australia: Cengage Learning.

Goleman, D. 2006. *Social intelligence: The new science of human relationships*. New York: Bantam Dell.

Grint, K., and C. Holt. 2011. *Followership in the NHS*. London: The Kings Fund. http://www. kingsfund.org.uk/sites/files/kf/followership-in-nhs-commississon-on-leadership-Management-keith-grint-claire-holt-kings-fund-may-2011.pdf.

Handy, C. 2000. *21 ideas for managers*. San Francisco: Jossey-Bass.

Kaplan, A. M., and M. Haenlin. 2010. Users of the world, unite! The challenges and opportunities of social media. *Business Horizons* 53: 59–68.

Kelley, R. E. 1992. *The power of followership*. New York: Currency.

Kings Fund 2011. *The future of leadership and management in the NHS: No more heroes*. London, England: The Kings Fund. http://www.kingsfund.org.uk/publications/future-leadership-and-management-nhs.

Lencioni, P. 2002. *The five dysfunctions of a team: A leadership fable*. San Francisco: Jossey Bass.

Lovegrove, M., and P. Long. 2012. Are radiographers prepared for the clinical leadership challenge? *Radiography* 18 (4): 230–31.

Luft, J. 1984. *Group processes: An introduction to group dynamics*, 3rd ed. Palo Alto, CA: Mayfield.

McCrindle Research. 2013. *Australia: The digital media nation report*. http://www.mccrindle.com. au/the-mccrindle-blog/australia-the-digital-media-nation

Miller, J. D. 2011. Active, balanced and happy: These young Americans aren't bowling alone. *The Generation X Report* 1 (1): 1–8. http://lsay.org/GenX_Rept_Iss1.pdf.

Shao, G. 2009. Understanding the appeal of user-generated media: A uses and gratification perspective. *Internet Research* 19 (1): 7–25.

Sivers, D. 2010. *How to start a movement*. http://www.ted.com/talks/derek_sivers_how_to_start_a_movement.html.

# 6 Effective Leadership of Teams

Sue Mellor

## Introduction

This chapter endeavours to reignite and stimulate your excellence and encourages you to draw on your experiences with teams. It addresses some basic concepts, offers ideas for your consideration and provides practical tools to support continuous team development, extending the concept of followership in Chapter 5 and drawing on a strong sense of self-awareness (Chapter 2).

Leading teams through the complexity of modern healthcare systems can be challenging and requires authentic leadership. Team membership may change on a daily basis, but your compassion, integrity and the other elements of your leadership, which remain constant, can make a better team than you may have ever thought possible.

Trust your inner leader and be brave!

Let's start with you.

## REFLECTION

- Do you consider yourself to be a team player?
- What are the implications of your answer to the previous question?
- What are the challenges you face as a team leader?
- Do you trust your team to achieve?

Effective teams interact together—with synergy, trust and respect being amongst the foundations of their life force—to outperform teams who do not invest in these qualities. A team is something that is put together, but it is how a team works together that will define their effectiveness.

There are some pre-requisites for optimal team performance; agreeing on the team's purpose, clarifying roles and responsibilities and defining values, goals and strategy are of major importance, but the group effort can be scuppered if the team does not exhibit professional values and behaviours. The complexity for the team leader is that we all have slightly different interpretations of behavioural norms. It may be acceptable to swear on some building sites but not so in a hospital clinic.

Not everyone is a natural team player, and that is OK. They can still offer a valuable contribution when they feel respected and appreciated, so long as they exhibit acceptable professional behaviour and are clear on the role expected of them. Have you ever agreed what are considered acceptable behaviours?

## Team-Building Events

Development of teams rarely just happens. Taking time out of the workplace to talk and listen to each other beyond basic work exchanges is beneficial to building team relationships. Hawkins (2011, p. 54) notes that team development is often initially focussed on the team's 'boundaries, membership and rules'.

Team building appears to be metamorphosing from a bonding event—often for a newly formed team, designed to draw the members together—to more recently including some of the features outlined in the following discussion. Often it's only an annual event, facilitated by an external consultant, which may incur a cost, so team members are required to learn from that expertise and integrate that learning into their everyday working. They are expected to develop a natural, dynamic and ongoing process, often without appropriate follow-up support.

The common ambitions of a team-building event clarify:

- What is the core business of your team?
- What are the team's goals?
- When measured against team goals, how well do individuals perform?
- What are the challenges being faced and how can they be overcome?
- How can the team work even more efficiently and effectively?
- What do we expect from each other, often from the perspective of support, trust, and loyalty?

Common issues raised include:

- The need for better communication
- A lack of clarity regarding values, goals, priorities and who is responsible for what
- A request for more resources (Sometimes they do need more, and sometimes there are opportunities for working smarter.)
- The need for support to manage conflict

## REFLECTION

- If you were to prepare a team-building day for your team, what would your ideal list of topics include?

- What would having input on each of those topics give the team?

Whilst having an annual event with a good facilitator can provide years of stories, the impact on performance unfortunately can be short term. Consider the last team-building event you attended: What was discussed and agreed, and is that still progressing? What support could have been provided that might have extended that ongoing learning?

Utilising an expert team-building facilitator can provide great benefits. However, many teams can make incremental steps on a regular basis by deliberately focusing on and developing the team, alongside the day-to-day provision of services, and by having clear outcomes in mind and an action plan the whole team 'owns'.

### SHORT STORY

A team exercise on the first floor of a venue: two teams had to get their team members from one side of the room to the other across obstacles. We later debriefed. During debrief the participants were asked if anyone had cheated in any way. All denied cheating; they even became agitated they were being questioned. Two 'mature' ladies did eventually admit that they had actually left the room, gone down one set of stairs, across the ground floor and back up another set of stairs to enter the room at the task end. We had an interesting conversation about creativity and rule bending.

## REFLECTION

- What learning can be taken from this story?

- What thoughts arise about your (and individual members'), values/rules/policies/flexibility?

- How might that differ between colleagues?

# Simple Ideas to Develop Teams In-House

1. *Using a quiz to develop knowledge*: Develop a 5-minute quiz for the next team meeting that includes questions relevant to the team's learning needs. It's a good way of developing knowledge in a non-threatening manner and a fun team tool.

## ACTIVITY

### Know Your Organisation

Create two teams: how is not important; it is just fun.

With a pen and paper, ask them 10 questions that are relevant and that they should perhaps know. In this example related to knowing your organisation, you could be creative with the topics you choose.

#### Examples

- What is the name of the CEO/chief nurse?
- What is the name of the medical director?
- Name one award recently won by a team in the hospital.
- What is our team's annual stationery/pharmacy/investigations budget?
- What are the top three compliments we receive from patient feedback?
- When are the policies due for review?
- How long is our patient waiting list?
- How many people are in the team (did you include the cleaner, night staff, etc?)
- Who in the team:

  Is related to someone famous?

  Has an interesting or unusual skill/hobby?

Remember that such a quiz is a shared exercise to enhance the team and that no individual should ever feel exposed.

2. *Social events*: This could be anything that appeals to your team, for example: attending a health spa together, a pub quiz, tai chi or bringing in cakes for birthdays.

   Be sensitive that not all members may want to take part—and that is OK! Consider how to make those not involved still feel included. Try to pick something that appeals to them next time. Also be sensitive to personal circumstances, such as caring responsibilities or possible financial constraints that may restrict participation.

3. *Fundraising*: A great way to bring people together is to support a cause with some link or importance to the team. This could be championing the hospital or possibly to raise funds for your own patients. Again, remember that not everyone may want to take part, so be respectful to their decision, but do ensure that everyone is invited and welcome. Fundraising can have the added benefit of developing wider networks and opportunities for shared projects in the future.

4. *Taking a team from average to excellence*: Teams who have annual team-building events may consider developing an annual team 'appraisal' into

the process. This can be achieved using the principles of staff appraisal, even using a similar formula so that members are familiar with the format. Ensure the team reviews their values, goals and purpose, how they work well together, and, importantly, how that rapport could be further improved. Ask them about their individual strengths that contribute to and develop the team whilst identifying training needs.

By reviewing accomplishment for the previous year, they can agree on the strategy for the forthcoming year, celebrate team achievements, and acknowledge success, in addition to ensuring their accomplishments.

## Team Feedback for the Brave

Teams in health care are interdependent on each other to provide a complex array of services that contribute to patient outcomes.

Extra-brave leaders could ask other departments with whom they regularly interact to provide constructive feedback regarding what their team does well and identify improvement opportunities to enhance synergy in the patient pathway. As the team leader, you need to analyse the feedback to ensure that it is valid, constructive and helpful to improving your team's performance.

This can improve relationships with other teams, as they may feel that their opinion is valued and well regarded.

## The Personal Specification Exercise

When we advertise a job, we review the competencies required and personal attributes desired (for example, team worker/good communicator).

### ACTIVITY

Assume that a post in your team is to be advertised.

Ask the team to agree about the personal qualities required to become a member of the team (ensure that they are specific).

Generate a team list.

Ask each member to *silently* reflect the score they attribute to themselves for each of the qualities.

The characteristics they have identified will give you insight as to what they deem important and provide an indication of their team values. You can explore with the team how those attributes are currently demonstrated and where they could be further enhanced.

## Learning Together

Learning together can be a great way to develop deeper team rapport. We often don't get a chance to talk about things that matter to us at work.

You may have noticed that those who get on well together are often seen together at breaks, etc. You can provide that opportunity to enhance team rapport by inviting guest speakers into team training, or sending team members together on mandatory training sessions, where possible, and asking them to feedback top tips to the team on their return. This may also provide enhanced application of their learning when they return to the clinical environment, giving even greater return on investment.

## Summary

Remember, as a leader you cannot cover everything on this list (at least not all in one year!). Select the activities that appeal to your team and that you believe will most effectively meet their needs. After any activity, take time to reflect on what was effective and what value each element had, so you know if they are worth using again in the future. Your role as a leader is to look at ways you can build, grow, empower and engage your team on an ongoing basis. You are building your team's identity (see the following section). Do it deliberately and with respect for each person who plays a part. Involve your team in deciding what activities they would like to see supported.

# So What Is Team Identity?

Think about sporting teams: they tend to wear specific colours or a sports kit; think of the armed forces, who pride themselves on the uniforms that identify the service they belong to. Many teams have a song uniting the supporters; others demonstrate rituals, like the All Blacks rugby team doing the Haka prior to each game. There are numerous indications of healthcare team identity from professional badges, uniforms, team languages, abbreviations and symbols.

## REFLECTION

- What identifies you as part of your team?
- Is that what you want to be identified by?
- If not, how would you prefer to be identified and what can you do about that?

In health care, staff often belong to professional bodies and even introduce themselves through their professional discipline. We are now seeing the benefits of developing multi-professional teams, especially regarding disease-specific teams, managing care across care pathways. Members often belong to more than one team: their professional body and their clinical team. These relationships become fluid over time, with individuals moving between teams regularly and boundaries between disciplines blurring as professionals work together to ensure excellence in patient care. It is worth considering how both teams and individuals retain an identity and the possible effect of those changing dynamics.

## REFLECTION

- List the different teams you are a member of.
- How would you describe the identity of each of those teams?
- How would others describe the team? What positive (or even negative) things would they note?
- How does your behaviour change in different teams/roles within a team?
- What could you do to build team identity further? Indeed, do you consider team identity to be a valuable entity?

## Let's Explore Why Team Identity Is Important

People take pride in belonging to something they value and have loyalty to their colleagues and team. It is even suggested that human beings have a need to belong. They enjoy being a part of something that contributes either to their own lives like a family or to a team that makes a difference. We naturally enjoy being a part of something we believe in and perceive to be performing well.

This is particularly common for those in health care, who recognise that their performance impacts directly or indirectly on the patient experience. We believe that membership in a team that works well together can provide satisfaction and a sense of well-being and belonging. Team identity can promote team cohesiveness and interdependence. Katzenbach and Smith (1993, 109) discuss the importance of developing trust within a team to support the journey from individual to mutual accountability, as only then do we see a really cohesive team.

If we explore feedback to teams, it is important for positive progress to be reflected to the team. Feedback is an opportunity to understand what we do well but also to further develop our identity. Developing a history together helps a team to develop its identity.

## REFLECTION

- When your team is at their very best, how would you describe it?
- What are they doing that creates excellence?
- How do others describe the team when it's most effective and harmonious?

# Highly Effective Teams

We work in teams because we cannot expect an individual to have all the required attributes, competencies and skills and because we can achieve more together than we can as individuals. That can be translated into solid returns that can be measured. West (2004, p. 18) notes that effective teams are not only more productive, but have personal benefits for the team members too, including lower stress levels.

Leading teams through change and ambiguity requires leaders to be flexible and reflexive to the needs of the situation and of those involved. However, it is worth the effort because, as Katzenbach and Smith (1993, p. 15) note, 'teams and performance are an unbeatable combination'.

## REFLECTION

Consider the most effective team you have ever been a member of.

- What was it about that team that made it so effective? Capture the key words that embody the team's characteristics.

- How can you begin to introduce even more of that into your current team?

There are many seminal texts that offer guidance to leaders about the fundamentals of effective teams, yet with a little reflective time, you will realise how much you already know intuitively.

Effective teams usually have some core characteristics. Often, phrases such as 'We knew what we were there to do'; 'We supported each other'; 'Everyone knew what was expected of them'; and 'We communicated'. (How many of those appeared on your list when reflecting on when your team was working well?)

It could be easily argued that within health care we have not just effective teams, but teams who work effectively across professional boundaries. Think about the journey the average patient takes through health care and the range of healthcare professionals the patient comes into contact with. Each individual and team is dependent on those who came into contact with the patient before and after them; how they interrelate supports a patient's seamless care pathway. (Chapter 7 will explore the shifting boundaries of healthcare teams in more depth.)

The inspirational, collaborative, authentic leader with natural insight is instrumental to a team's success, and well-defined goals that are challenging yet realistic are a prerequisite for an effective team. You can only measure your success if you know what it is going to look, feel and sound like (emphasising again the importance of having a clear vision, as discussed in Chapter 3, and of setting goals, a topic addressed in Chapter 14).

Let's explore some of the basic concepts of effective teams a little further:

## The Purpose of a Highly Effective Team

Team members need to understand where they fit in the organisational jigsaw and, importantly, what their purpose is as a team and how that impacts on the bigger picture. Within health care, that is often an easy task at a local level, as most of us recognise that our team plays one part in an elaborate labyrinth of a patients pathway. For many, this will be linked to their personal values and beliefs and therefore has their commitment. But, in addition, it requires members to take wider responsibility for their role to represent their team to ensure that their team performance contributes to the wider healthcare service delivery. It is sometimes this extra step that can be forgotten, which may impact on the whole patient experience.

## Communication Tips

Beyond any doubt, one of the most common elements flagged by teams in trouble includes communication. It would seem that no matter in how many different ways and however many times information is relayed, clear concise communication is beneficial. People have different ways of communicating and different needs; it is worth asking them to summarise back what you have said in order to ensure that the message sent was the same as the message received (we call this 'checking it out'). The art is to deliver the information in a manner that it is heard, understood and accepted even if not agreed with. (Communication is covered in more depth in Chapter 4.)

**REFLECTION**

Use a grid similar to Table 6.1 to make a list of your team members. Next to each one, consider the following heading for each:

**How does each individual like to be rewarded?**

Do they like to be thanked for their contribution in front of others so that their accomplishments are openly acknowledged, or do they prefer to see their name in a newsletter, or would they prefer a quiet coffee with the leader to discuss their achievements? Different people prefer different rewards; do not assume everyone is motivated by what motives you.

Remember, a kind word generates feelings of value, which lead to increased satisfaction, good will and engagement, a core aim for all teams. As the team leader, *you* may not need external validation, but your members might. Are you giving the right messages about being valued in a way they relate to? (And if you are not sure, just ask them. It shows how serious you are about wanting to recognise and value their preferences and contributions. It demonstrates a genuine interest in your colleagues.)

Highly Effective Teams

**Table 6.1** Grid

| Name | Strengths | Motivated by | Likes to be rewarded by | Learning needs | Responds to type of leadership style | Preferred learning style |
|------|-----------|--------------|-------------------------|----------------|--------------------------------------|--------------------------|
| Liz | Good communicator | Challenging targets | Verbal praise | Understanding Human Factors | Directive | Activist |
| | | | | | | |
| | | | | | | |
| | | | | | | |
| | | | | | | |

The leader who is aware of and flexible to the needs of individuals will inspire members, encouraging each to give their utmost for the team.

## Managing Membership Changes

It is a natural dynamic for team members to leave and new members to join. This can be challenging to the team synergy for all involved, and can even be disruptive at times as we develop new relationships and sometimes mourn the leaving of a teammate. It can also be a huge opportunity to build an even better team.

Introducing a new team member with a valuable contribution can provide new opportunities as the team reforms and evolves. Remember, a new team member will bring two things: previous experience that can offer some learning and 'fresh eyes'. Embraced as an opportunity whilst acknowledging that some may initially see it as a threat, both elements from the new member are useful to a team that wants to enhance their performance.

## Team Meetings to Support Team Communication

Ask a team what they need to improve; communication is always near the top of the list. Regular team meetings often go by the wayside as things get busier. Actually, that is when you need them the most. Team meetings offer the opportunity to build relationships, confirm team direction, reevaluate immediate team goals, prioritise actions and clarify who is responsible for what, and evaluate and celebrate progress. That can include developing opportunities for creativity. Get into the habit of asking team members big, open questions: 'What can we improve even further?' and 'What are we doing well?' and 'What problems are we still tackling?'

These questions may at first seem to elicit few responses. However, as the leader evidences his or her commitment to improvement through listening and possibly piloting some of the ideas, members will become more courageous in engaging in the ongoing conversation, and innovative opportunities can follow. A 5-minute briefing at shift change for the sake of wider situational awareness can also enhance communication and safety.

## Roles and Responsibilities

Clarifying roles and responsibilities is fundamental for effective teams, without which elements of confusion and duplication of roles can lead to conflict.

Asking members to share changes in their responsibilities at the team meeting can ensure that team members are aware of new perspectives. It also provides a platform for others to offer assistance so that relevant information may be shared, affording wider team ownership.

## Conflict in Teams: 'A Conflict Splinter'

It is worth saying that some conflict is normal. It can range from a small transient disagreement to a full-blown angry fallout with long-term ramifications. The art is for the leader to identify whether it is simply a small 'splinter' that will naturally heal and relates to healthy discussions, which may even strengthen relationships (West 2004, 8), or if it may be a 'splinter' that might become infected if not dealt with, potentially infecting the whole team over time.

Early support is key to combating destructive conflict. If you are concerned, checking your options is a wise thing to do; even if you then decide to do nothing, at least you will have made an informed choice. Often it is better to tackle an issue when it is a splinter that can be easily resolved, not waiting for it to become a fully grown infection. Executive coaching can help you work through the issues to identify your options in a safe 'test' environment and help you define the skills to handle the conflict effectively back in the team context.

Alternatively, your supervisor, mentor, manager, human resource team or an organisational improvement team can help you explore the dynamics of the conflict and offer appropriate support, ensuring that you work within any workplace policy and procedures.

The skilled leader ensures that each perspective is valued, and members feel that their views are respected.

# Communicating and Sharing the Vision

We can work in teams for years and not reflect again on the basics of why we are there, together, as a team. It is often assumed that we all had (and have) the same vision and sense of responsibility towards organisational goals. Verbalising the vision, at least on an annual basis, ensures that everyone is going in the same direction and reminds individuals of their overall purpose in the team.

## ACTIVITY

Ask each member of your team to write in no more than three sentences the vision for the team and separately the purpose of the team. Ask them to read them out without questions from colleagues other than those for clarification.

Use this as an opportunity to clarify the direction of the team and to develop a joint understanding whilst recognising we all see things slightly differently and have different ways of communicating our messages.

Taking the time to confirm a clear vision in everyone's mind, as well as how they contribute to the overall outcome, should provide a sense of interdependence, belonging and respect for different perspectives. There is usually some clear common ground, and in health care it often links to making a difference to the patient experience.

A written team pledge is often a good visual reminder.

# Prioritise

Clarifying roles and responsibilities together with the team's overall priorities facilitates effective management of team workloads. Understanding individual members' priorities and how their progress contributes to the wider team is also valuable to understand. It provides the opportunity to support each other, either by sharing information that is pertinent or through redistribution of work if required to enable the team goals to be met. A simple urgent/soon or routine label attributed to each task can be constructive and prevent the team from feeling overwhelmed.

# On the Road to Excellence

At your team meetings, remember the importance of sharing what is expected of all the team and its members. This can be anything from implementing a new process, reviewing a new system, celebrating success or ensuring that the whole team is trained on a new piece of equipment.

## ACTIVITY

Ask each member to:

- Identify their top three priorities for the week/month ahead
- Clarify how they are progressing and what is going well
- Identify any challenges or barriers they are facing
- Identify areas where they need help or support (as well as where such support could come from)
- Generate new ideas around what may improve the patient experience

It is amazing how team members will pull together if they recognise the impact on the team of not reaching their goals/objectives. They will often help each other, which builds good will in the team's 'bank of support'.

## Team Resilience

The pace of change is phenomenal in health care; as science progresses, technology follows, and the quest to be cost effective is becoming a team responsibility (while still ensuring excellent high quality patient care). Like a tree that can bend in the wind, the team that can respond to the changing healthcare landscape—indeed, the team that expects a constantly changing landscape—is more likely to deal effectively with the challenges they face.

The needs of individuals in the team will differ, and the team needs to be reflexive in the support it provides each member and be honest regarding their needs of each other. The best leaders flex to the needs of the individuals whilst remaining vigilant to the team purpose and keeping the goal in sight.

## Expectations of Each Other in the Team

Managing expectations of each other is a helpful way of ensuring that team members have an agreement of what is expected of them. We all have behaviours identified that we consider acceptable when working together, yet we have all seen and possibly even displayed (if we are honest) behaviours that are not optimal. Developing the rules within the team so that people know when they are stepping over the line helps towards building trust. Trust is built and based often on experience, and once broken, it can be extremely difficult to rebuild. Therefore, taking the time to identify what the team considers acceptable and unacceptable (and how that can be handled) will help to build trust.

## REFLECTION

For evidence of this, think of a time when someone has behaved in an unacceptable manner and the impact it has had on the team. What was handled well? What could have been handled even better (and how)?

## Whatever the Function of Your Team: A Last Thought

As a team leader, your focus is on delivering or supporting the delivery of excellence in patient care, and your role is to facilitate that through your team. You may not be hands-on with a patient directly, but you can always be supporting someone who is. You have a dual role: to do your own role excellently, ensuring self-leadership and effectiveness, and in addition, you have a key role in empowering each individual in your team to reach their potential so that they can contribute fully to team goals. It is a huge responsibility, but also an incredible privilege. We hope this chapter helps you to be even more effective at it in the future.

## References

Hawkins, P. 2011. *Leadership team coaching*. London: Kogan Page.
Katzenbach, J., and D. Smith. 1993. *The wisdom of teams*. Berkshire: McGraw-Hill.
West, M. 2004. *The secrets of successful team management*. London: Duncan Baird.

## Recommended Reading

The Clinical Human Factors Group, www.chfg.org.

# 7 Leading in Health Care: Challenging Boundaries and Future Potential

Maryann Hardy, Bev Snaith and Suzanne Henwood

Now that you have looked at teams, this chapter will explore the wider and strategic leadership issues and some of the challenges related to changing team boundaries and disciplines coming together to improve patient care through collaborative patient services across the care pathway.

## Drivers for Changing Roles in Health Care

Public interest worldwide in healthcare availability, quality and new treatments as well as healthy living has grown rapidly over the last 30 years. Illness and disease are no longer perceived to be the inevitable consequence of living but, instead, are viewed as preventable or treatable phenomena. As a result, public expectations of healthcare systems and healthcare professionals have changed beyond the sterile routine of hospital and primary-care regimes dominated by medical leadership. Instead, with the help of easy-to-access information, predominantly through Internet sources, increasingly informed populations demand to be more involved in healthcare decision making and insist on clear explanations for treatment choices and rehabilitation regimes.

Of course globally the position of different cultural societies is not identical. Variations in healthcare provision and access to health care are clearly dependent on the economic wealth of the country and region as well as the prevailing health service culture, which may be dominated by social or private enterprise. However, what is clear is that the economics of health care as well as clear evidence as to the success of interventions are global priorities. It is this drive for cost-effective healthcare provision that was one of the drivers behind the need for evidence-based medicine

(Sackett et al. 1996), subsequently abridged to evidence-based practice to encompass nursing and allied health professionals.

## Questioning Traditional Healthcare Roles

At the same time as healthcare providers were placing financial restrictions on service provision and treatment availability, research priorities globally were changing, with emphasis being placed on doing more with less or maximising the use of scarce health resources. Common to all healthcare systems is that the most expensive resource is staff, in particular medical staff. Consequently, questions began to be asked of the role of medical staff and whether some of these roles could be undertaken by other staff groups. How might advancing computer technology support remote medical consultation? Could tele-consultation be used to support a non-medical–led intervention, particularly in rural or sparsely inhabited areas?

This change in strategic thinking around healthcare provision questioned the absolute practice boundaries developed by individual professional groups, in particular medicine, and overtly promoted, perhaps for the first time, the autonomy and capability of non-medical health professions in healthcare decision making. Importantly, the crucial factor in this change in strategic thinking, and the catalyst for the accelerated adoption of new ways of working, was the development of outcomes-focussed healthcare practices. Societal research was demonstrating clearly the negative economic and social impact of ill health and disease. Therefore, healthcare services needed to ensure that early and appropriate intervention was implemented to minimise the long-term effects of ill health and, more importantly, engage communities in healthy living activities. To support this, services started to be restructured around the needs of the patient rather than trying to force patient pathways into existing service-delivery models. To ensure the success of these new models of care, the need for non-medical staff to take on new roles became apparent.

## REFLECTION

Think about the service you and your organisation provides:

1. How do patients access the service? Are there long delays in initial diagnosis and treatment? What factors influence this? What impact do you see this having on society as a whole?

2. Is the service designed to meet the requirement of the organisation (e.g., limited to daytime operation), or is the service available at a time that best suits the patient (e.g., evenings, weekends)?

3. Do patients on a treatment pathway have to attend the clinic/hospital on several different occasions for investigation or treatment (e.g., medical consultation, imaging, blood tests, physiotherapy), or are the appointments

streamlined to minimise disruption to the patient and their family? How might a more streamlined approach also benefit the different health specialities?

4. What would the patient see as a high-quality health service? Would this be different to their view of your organisation currently?

Consider these questions and identify where improvement might be made and what interventions might be necessary to accomplish change. What are the key barriers to change, and who could positively influence taking changes forward? How could such changes be evaluated: when and by whom?

## Role Extension, Expansion, Advancement, Delegation and Substitution: The UK Experience

Much healthcare professional literature has explored the extension, expansion and advancement of non-medical roles (the terms being used synonymously within this chapter) as a consequence of the opportunities to develop outcome-driven patient services in response to new interventions, treatments and diagnostic technologies. While international interest exists in the extension, expansion and advancement of non-medical roles, many of these new roles include tasks previously undertaken by medical practitioners, and therefore their successful implementation is in many ways reliant on the willingness of medical practitioners to delegate responsibility for specific tasks to wider healthcare professional groups. It is perhaps useful at this point, then, to consider the development of non-medical role extension in the United Kingdom (UK) as an example of a country where autonomous advanced practice and role extension has been widely, though inconsistently, implemented.

The UK is unique in the Western world in providing social health care that is free at the point of access (National Health Service [NHS]). As a result, healthcare provision is predominantly funded by the government supported through a system of national contribution akin to taxation. While the potential opportunities for role extension of the non-medical professions had been discussed in many UK fora during the 1990s and earlier, the real facilitator of change was the government's vision for an updated health service. This included the introduction of a new national staff grading and pay structure (Agenda for Change) that included advanced and consultant practice roles for nurses and allied health professions. It needs to be emphasised that while pockets of advanced and extended role evolution were occurring across the UK throughout the 1990s, this was ad hoc and locally driven. Government policy was central to changing the way individual professions viewed themselves, and each other, and the new grading structure ensured that the development of advanced non-medical roles was taken seriously, recognising the contribution of the multiple, essential and talented professions within the health service in realising the government's vision. As a result, health professionals were encouraged to move away from traditional and hierarchical working practices and to work together at all levels of practice to improve patient pathways and experience through shared models of multidisciplinary leadership and service provision.

These changes in UK healthcare service provision represented a significant culture shift in terms of management and leadership within the NHS. The UK government was calling for a distributive team approach to leadership, with all professions and patients being involved in decision making as opposed to previous individualistic leadership approaches (transactional or transformational), which were dependent as much on the charisma and personality of the individual as the strategic direction and goals of the organisation (Currie and Lockett 2011; Graham and Learmonth 2012). Interestingly, while the government was promoting patient-centred care, cost-efficiency, improvements in clinical quality and patient outcomes and the expansion of the role of clinicians in driving forward change, the role of managers and administrators, who had previously been responsible for guiding service provision and "balancing the books" in terms of cost, appeared to take a back seat. As a result, their influence and contribution to decision making was felt by some to be diminished, resulting in some organisations restructuring management roles.

## REFLECTION

Consider the political and public agenda in terms of health care within your own country:

1. What is the vision of health care going forwards? What do healthcare providers (private and public) aim to achieve?

2. How might role extension, expansion and advancement within the non-medical professions enable these aims to be achieved?

3. What is driving such changes? Is there clear clinical need and benefit to patients?

4. How might changes in how you and your professional group practise impact on service costs and efficiency, including impact on patient outcomes and patient experience?

The argument for the delegation of medical roles, normally involving routine tasks, to nurses and allied health professionals was that this would allow medical practitioners to concentrate on the more difficult cases requiring medical decision making rather than routine or standard care that, by its nature of being routine, could be delivered by non-medical professionals through protocol-driven processes. The anticipated outcome of this initiative was that more people could receive prompt appropriate care, thereby reducing costs and increasing service efficiency without compromising patient outcomes.

Understandably, while many nurses and allied health professionals welcomed the opportunity to extend their roles and make a greater contribution to patient pathways, the changes to non-medical roles threatened some medical professionals. Medical personnel argued that to place full autonomy, accountability and responsibility for (medical) decision making within the role of a non-medical professional presented significant clinical risk. They suggested instead that the non-medical professional should not work in isolation, but instead should be part of a clinical team led by a medical practitioner who would delegate appropriate duties. The medical practitioner would also be responsible for auditing the practice of the non-medical professional to ensure that standards were being maintained.

This appeared to be an appropriate and supportive delivery structure that was readily agreed to by all parties. However, in practice, this has meant that professional autonomy to drive forward service change has, in many cases, been restricted by medical colleagues being unwilling to relinquish routine roles. Importantly, this has also impacted on research into this field, with published studies focussing predominantly on establishing the competencies of non-medical health professionals wishing to extend their role rather than evaluating how the incorporation of extended, advanced or specialist non-medical roles have impacted on service quality, efficiency and patient outcomes. Indeed, Humphreys et al. (2007), in their systematic review to evaluate the effectiveness of nurse, midwife and allied health professional consultant roles, conclude that 'the extent to which these roles "add value" and provide cost-effectiveness has not yet been evaluated'. Further, Humphreys et al. state that the 'assessment of impact is complex particularly where roles have been operationalised in different ways and affect different services and care'. This is an important learning point for international colleagues wishing to implement advanced-practice roles, a topic that is explored later in this chapter.

Because the system of introducing advanced-practice roles in the UK was reliant on medical responsibility and accountability for task delegation, no consistent model of advanced practice was developed. The Agenda for Change framework did determine the generic criteria for advanced practice, but these were interpreted differently across the country and, as a result, local variation in non-medical roles and responsibilities occurred based upon the willingness of individual medical practitioners to delegate roles (Lloyd Jones 2005). On reflection, this is in part because the registerable title of the non-medical health profession in the UK relates to threshold first-post competencies and not advanced roles beyond initial registration. As a result, there is no national register of advanced-competency personnel, although many professional bodies provide voluntary accreditation for advanced and consultant practice. Further, as delegation of duties often requires support of a medical practitioner within the employing organisation, the mobility of staff with extended roles across health organisations (even just in the UK) has been restricted, as medical support for role extension in one organisation may not be forthcoming in another.

Interestingly, it appears that a similar pattern is emerging in the United States in terms of physician assistant or extender roles, although this variation in practice and limited mobility may be as much to do with the differences in healthcare systems and legislature across the states as professional delegation processes. There is also the issue of being able to 'charge' for physician-assistant activity, an important factor in private healthcare systems. Much discussion has occurred in relation to this between healthcare organisations and major health insurance providers, particularly in terms of a sliding scale of costs dependent on who is undertaking the work. Despite similar issues to the UK in terms of inconsistent implementation of advanced-practice roles, the USA has developed education programmes specifically aimed at developing physician assistants and role extenders within the different specialty areas with some content parity, which may permit greater staff mobility in the future. This again contrasts with the UK, where education for extended roles has been driven by the clinical tasks undertaken rather than the role itself, although it may be argued that the variety within masters-level education expected for advanced practice will provide opportunity to learn wider skills.

A final example of implementation strategy for advanced practice can be taken from the radiography professional body in Australia (Australian Institute of Radiography) who, in collaboration with medical radiologist professional organisations, have developed a national programme for radiography advanced practice to ensure transparency and equity in role opportunity, expectations and development. While at the time of writing this chapter it seemed that this strategy was on the verge of implementation (Freckelton 2012), it appears from the strategy document that some evaluation of existing international implementation experiences has been undertaken to inform the development of a nationally agreed strategy.

## Application to Practice

It is evident that while international interest in non-medical role development exists, the process of developing and implementing these roles varies. However, we should keep in mind that the primary purpose of role extension is to improve healthcare service delivery and patient outcomes and experience within the context of local healthcare provision. That is, the priorities for healthcare intervention should be driven by organisational and population need and not individual professional gain.

It is important to stress that while this chapter has so far considered advanced-practice implementation and some of the issues that have been experienced, particularly in the UK, these have not been a barrier to professional leadership and service improvement initiatives. Instead, non-medical clinicians have found ways to address the barriers to development through collaboration, negotiation and, in some cases, doggedly pursuing their service improvement ideals.

Below are examples of such advanced practice roles within nursing and allied health professions in the UK and how they contribute to health service delivery. The remainder of the chapter will present some thoughts to encourage deeper reflection on a range of opportunities and challenges for those wanting to lead change and become, or implement, advanced-practice roles, which may challenge existing roles and team boundaries. However, it must be stressed that role development and professional leadership in health care are dynamic entities, and these points reflect the authors' thoughts at the time of writing and are in no way all-encompassing or exhaustive but are intended to be thought provoking. We would ask you as the reader to relate the examples here to your own organisational context to explore what learning is possible and relevant to your own practice area.

## Advanced Practice Role Examples

### Nurse

Karl is a nurse who works as part of a team delivering primary-care services alongside general practitioners. He runs asthma and smoking-cessation clinics as well as contributing to weekly drop-in clinics and is extending his role to undertake supplementary prescribing. His role provides extended practice skills within a wider team.

### Nurse

Helen has worked within gynaecology since qualifying as a nurse in 1990 and has a particular interest in empowering women from disadvantaged or culturally diverse backgrounds to access women's health services. Alongside others, Helen developed the outpatient hysteroscopy service, where her role includes management of the facilities, triage of referrals, history taking, diagnosis and treatment, debriefing, referring on and attending multi-disciplinary meetings, and auditing outcomes against national standards. She is currently the only nurse in the UK to have completed the postgraduate diploma in gynaecology for health professionals with a special interest and is involved in nurse and medical training and examining in this field. She is on the editorial board of the *Primary Care Women's Health Journal*, for which she writes regularly, and she and her team have been recognised for their innovative work through a number of national award schemes.

### Radiographer

Beverly is a consultant radiographer in emergency care. She has extended her clinical skills to include image reporting as well as ultrasound scanning and reporting. Alongside her own role development, she has led and implemented practice changes in imaging and emergency care. As a consultant, her leadership is strategic rather than operational and is focussed on improving patient care at the forefront of the evidence base.

### Physiotherapist

Colin is an extended-scope physiotherapy practitioner specialising in musculoskeletal lower-limb conditions. His extended role includes referring for imaging investigations, including X-rays, MRI and ultrasound scans, to assist in planning treatment and interventions. He has also completed a course allowing him to perform soft-tissue and joint injections. In addition to his clinical role, Colin works as a lecturer at the local university. His role as an expert practitioner enhances both the service and the work of others within the multidisciplinary orthopaedic team.

## REFLECTION

Consider the role of your own profession within your own country and internationally:

1. How has your profession changed over the last 20 years? What new roles has it taken on, and which of those are now encompassed in the standard scope of practice, and which are reserved for those staff working at a higher level clinically? What impact has this had on traditional role or team boundaries?

2. If you think ahead 10–20 years, where would you like to see your profession? What new ways of working, or new roles not yet in place, do you want to see established? What is needed to achieve this?

3. As an individual professional and leader, what part can you play (and will you play) in making the changes identified above happen? Try developing an action plan with short-, medium- and long-term targets and reflect on these often to identify your progress towards them. Consider who you need to liaise with, who can influence these developments and what first steps you can take to begin the discussions about making that happen.

# Thoughts on Opportunities for Change and Leadership Development

## Consumer-Driven Health Care

In many Western cultures, patients and service users are increasingly informed about the quality of services provided with a 'league table' culture prevailing. Service users are welcomed as informed consumers of health care to contribute to organisational governance structures. Importantly, the patient and service-user voice is being used to guide service improvements and operational changes and, as a result, the profile of non-medical healthcare practitioners is reported to be increasing. As private- and public-sector healthcare providers want their patient services to be viewed positively, professional developments that support patient empowerment and improve their healthcare experience are an important aspect of modern healthcare systems and an area where non-medical leadership and service-change activity can really develop without direct medical intervention.

### REFLECTION

With reference to your own professional practice:

1. How do patients describe a high-quality service? Is your service meeting their expectations? How do you measure patient satisfaction or gain service-user input into service design? What could you do to make this even more effective?

2. What service changes are required to improve patient satisfaction? How will these changes impact on other professional groups and services? Is there opportunity for collaboration and leadership in service change? Who do you need to work with and how will you begin to put in place that collaboration?

## Preferred-Care Setting

Specialist medical practitioners, particularly senior and consultant doctors, are an expensive resource and in order to be most cost effective, they need to be positioned where their expertise can be best utilised. Consequently, with the exception of general practitioners (GPs), most medical specialists are situated within secondary- or tertiary-care centres where specialist teams act as clinical experts. While some specialist physicians may offer peripatetic clinics within semi-urban centres, community health care in more rural environments is often limited. Even in urban suburbs, patients are demanding that routine care in particular be undertaken within their home or community environment. Non-medical specialists could evaluate routine procedures in their own area of practice and suggest alternative service-delivery patterns that better meet the demands of the service-user groups. Consideration also needs to be made of hard-to-reach (often minority) population groups or those who present late for diagnosis and treatment to help to address priorities in tackling population health inequalities. Within this changing health context, it may be useful to further develop non-medical referral and prescribing practices.

## Inter-Professional Blurred-Boundary Working

Blurred-boundary working is developing pace in the UK as a way of professions sharing responsibilities and roles in certain aspects of patient care in order to streamline services. For example, an elderly patient being discharged home after a fall may need to be seen by a physiotherapist to explain exercise therapy, an occupational therapist to look at behaviour modification and equipment to support and encourage independent living, a social worker to look at family support and additional social support necessary and a community nurse to ensure that wounds and dressing care can be maintained. In this situation, being seen by multiple practitioners may create confusion, especially where questions and advice appear similar. Would it not be better, therefore, for one person, who is appropriately trained, to be able to meet and assess the patient pre-discharge from the perspective of physiotherapy, occupational therapy, social work and community nursing? This sharing of responsibility at the professional boundaries is beginning to change the way we work, but it is at its early stages and has yet to be evaluated fully.

## Globalisation of Health Care

In the earlier part of this chapter, we mentioned the issues that have occurred with local role-development initiatives and resultant staff mobility restrictions for those working in advanced roles. However, now consider this on a global scale. Global migration (immigration and emigration) informs population diversity and priorities in health care going forwards. However, what is less clear is how an experienced healthcare practitioner undertaking an advanced-practice role with positive patient benefits in one part of the world can continue to use these skills for the benefit of patients within different healthcare systems should they move to another part of the world.

Many countries have addressed issues of global migration for healthcare workers through recognition of professional qualifications, use of national threshold practice examinations and skills-support programmes. But, if we are to make the best use of practitioner skills, is it time to recognise not only entry-level qualifications, but also advanced-practice roles globally? This is an area requiring strong and dynamic professional leadership. Telemedicine has meant that international partnerships exist in the delivery of medical decision making, but these have not been universally introduced with assessment of clinical skills, knowledge or cognisance of patient rights. In addition, the legal operating framework has been related to the country where the medical practitioner or telemedicine organisation is situated and not the country using the service (country of patient residence). Leadership to promote global cooperation and unified role developments among the nursing and allied health professions needs to be much more transparent. We would also argue that there is a need to promote sustainable and patient-focussed approaches to service delivery at the same time as considering the financial drivers for change.

## Impact of Technology on Health Care

We have previously mentioned the use of telemedicine within the context of global working. But the rapid advancement in technology has provided opportunities to improve services and change the way we work through its ongoing adaptation and implementation. Examples include patient-held electronic notes, electronic inter-agency referral and reporting procedures, handheld devices to support clinical decision making, patient booking services through social media and appointment reminders through phone text messaging, etc. Technology-enhanced learning is very much a part of most professional pre-registration curricula, but it is unclear how we incorporate these advances into practice and explore how they might benefit service provision and improve the patient experience. The important point here is that professional leaders are open to technological advancements and have the knowledge and skills to recognise their potential in service-improvement initiatives. What is less clear is how this is being incorporated and evaluated in practice to inform future learning opportunities.

## Developing the Research Evidence Base

As graduate professionals, it is an expectation that healthcare practitioners will be users of research and have the skills to critically appraise research findings in order to evidence research-informed practice. However, as leaders in service and practice development, many look to advanced and consultant practitioners to undertake the research that underpins this. Unfortunately, in published studies that have evaluated the role of advanced and consultant roles in the UK (Lloyd Jones 2005), while expert clinical practice skills are always seen as highly developed, research leadership is extremely weak. Perhaps this is because much effort has been put into demonstrating clinical competencies equivalent to our medical counterparts. Traditional research approaches have also been entrenched in the medical model of care and positivistic measures that are often unsuitable for research in non-medical fields. Finally, support and demand for the development of research skills has also been lacking from employers and staff alike, who fail to realise the relevance of research to evidence-based practice and leading service developments. While the number of non-medical healthcare professionals with research degrees (doctoral level) is small, it is increasing, although the majority appear to work within academia rather than clinical environments. We need to encourage this group of research-competent professionals to work with clinical practitioners to develop collaborative clinical-academic partnerships and use their combined knowledge to actively engage in research and inform the unique professional evidence base that underpins practice. Without a doubt, research expertise across all the non-medical professions is in need of leadership, and huge opportunities exist for multi-professional, multi-organisational and inter-continental collaboration.

## REFLECTION

What role do you and/or your department play in developing the research evidence base? What would be the first steps to making this even more effective?

One important consideration as you begin to engage more with global literature around changing professional boundaries is to critically review what you read and contextualise the language used. Titles such as 'consultant' are used very differently between professions and across the globe. For example, a consultant nurse in Australia has a very different status compared to a consultant nurse in the UK. There may also be significant confusion regarding the title among other professional groups and patients, especially where the term *consultant* implies a medical practitioner.

Research is already accumulating to evaluate the effectiveness of interventions in terms of patient outcomes and costs, but more is required to ensure sustainability of these roles into the future. Continuous audit and evidencing of effectiveness is important, but to prevent healthcare delivery systems reverting back to professional silos and protectionism, it may be that a new systems-based thinking approach is required (see Chapter 9).

## Summary

Any change and progress within moving role boundaries is set within a context, which has many components, including prevailing leadership culture and time frames. Much is written about historical medical dominance in health care, but recent literature shows a paradigm shift in healthcare leadership towards the need for collaboration, delegation and complex adaptive styles that are responsive to continuously changing and complex environments and problems.

In healthcare service delivery, we appear to be at a critical point in choosing how we wish to move forward. Are we ready to challenge long-established hierarchies and boundaries? Are we able to explore and test out new ways of working, which undoubtedly will cause some disruption to some and unsettle others? How do we develop 'new leaders'? Are we ready to embrace developments such as Action Learning Groups and Executive Coaching to enable people to step up into these new leadership roles? How do we identify and nurture future leaders and encourage the questioning of practice while ensuring maintenance of excellence in service delivery? How do we ensure that our future vision is shared by other professions, all of which are driving their own agendas?

Health care exists in a global, national and politically driven environment, and we have the responsibility to optimise patient health outcomes and population well-being while simultaneously making the best use of scarce resources. Now more than ever before we believe there is a requirement to build authentic, respectful relationships across professional boundaries and explore collaboratively (and with integrity) the best way of providing excellence in service provision into the future. What role will you play in creating that positive model of care locally? Nationally? And beyond? What is your first step to thinking and behaving differently?

## References

Currie, G., and A. Lockett. 2011. Distributing leadership in health and social care: concertive, conjoint or collective? *International Journal of Management Reviews* 13: 286–300.

Freckelton, I. 2012. *Advanced practise in radiography and radiation therapy: Report from an inrterprofessional advisory team*. Australian Institute of Radiography, Melbourne.

Graham, M. P., and M. Learmonth. 2012. A critical account of the rise and spread of 'leadership': The case of UK healthcare. *Social Science & Medicine* 74: 281–88.

Humphreys, A., S. Johnson, J. Richardson, E. Stenhouse, and M. Watkins. 2007. A systematic review and meta-synthesis: Evaluating the effectiveness of nurse, midwife and allied health professional consultants. *Journal of Clinical Nursing* 16 (10): 1792–1808.

Lloyd Jones, M. 2005. Role development and effective practise in specialist and advanced practise roles in acute hospital settings: Systematic review and meta-synthesis. *Journal of Advanced Nursing* 49 (2): 191–209.

Sackett, D. L., W. M. C. Rosenburg, J. A. M. Gray, R. B. Haynes, and W. S. Richardson. 1996. Evidence based medicine: What it is and what it isn't. *BMJ* 312: 71.

# 8 Leading and Change in Institutions

Joe Cheal and Melody Cheal

Any change of course sits within an organisational and/or institutional structure. In this chapter, we will be exploring the reasons for change and the role of the leader within a workplace context. We will give an overview of the context of organisational change and discuss what needs to be considered. Added to this, we will share with you some key ideas on how to encourage buy-in from stakeholders, management and staff.

## Why Change?

The nature of change is changing. Perhaps we could go one step further now in saying that the nature of change is accelerating. In the health service industry, the gap between changes is decreasing, and more changes are happening simultaneously or at least overlapping. One change is not yet in place before another layer of change is introduced.

Why the need for all this change? If things work okay, why not just leave them alone? Why risk interfering with what isn't broken? For the private sector, the answer is something along the lines of 'to be more competitive' and ultimately 'to make money'. However, in the public sector, a more likely answer is 'to be more efficient' and 'to save money'. The bad news is that the cost of *poorly considered* change tends to be greater than the money it saves. However, change does not have to be a difficult and lengthy process. By taking the time to think it through and getting buy-in at the beginning, change becomes an easier and smoother process for all involved.

# The Reasons for Change

Change tends to come about for three reasons (all of which are interconnected):

- *To solve a problem*: Something isn't working and needs to be fixed. Alternatively, there is a tension or dilemma of some kind that is creating a split or schism. The cost of a problem and its implications requires action to deal with it. This might be considered 'reactive' change.

- *To maintain or improve a situation*: Something needs maintaining, or perhaps it isn't great and could be better. Whilst it may not be broken, it might be tarnished in some way. Alternatively, there is a need to keep up with the environment (e.g., government policies, advances in technology, increases in standard of living). This might be considered 'responsive' change.

- *To achieve a goal*: There is an opportunity to be leading edge, to become the first to do something, to pioneer, to be at the top or to be number one. This might be considered 'proactive change'.

The first reason for change (i.e., to solve a problem) is usually the easiest to sell because it is more visible and affecting the system/people 'now'. However, it is about maintaining a status quo with *how things have been*. It does not necessarily account for the changing environment. We may well change to fix a problem, but this only brings us back to where we were before.

The second reason for change (i.e., to maintain or improve a situation) is a tougher sell because it is harder to see the immediate impact on the system/people. This type of change is about maintaining a status quo with *how things are now*. With a focus on the need for evidence in health care, research and compelling data will often be required. Sometimes we need to keep moving just to stay still! Of course, if this kind of situation is left unchecked, it will probably manifest as an overt problem, and then you are back to the first reason for change.

The third reason for change (i.e., to achieve a goal) is the toughest sell because it is about getting ahead of the environment. This type of change is about maintaining the status quo with *how things will be*. There usually needs to be a clear and visionary leader who is able to demonstrate evidence of how new initiatives are working. The benefits here need to be outstanding, because the cost of pioneering is usually expensive and potentially risky. If a hospital invests in 'experimental' research or equipment, there is a risk that that research will amount to nothing or the equipment will not deliver. In addition, tomorrow's knowledge and technology will be history once tomorrow passes.

In essence, as a leader, you will need to seek to stay current with responsive change (which will prevent some problems) and fix problems as they occur (reactive change). Regularly review the current state and the potential future, and then where necessary and possible, pioneer (proactive change). Of course, you will need to avoid making changes just for the sake of changing. There needs to be a reason and purpose for investing in change.

A recent NHS report (Neath 2009, p. 26) suggests that 'The most powerful change themes often have their origin in a dilemma.' This is where there is a belief that the organisation can do *either* one thing *or* another. The change is then designed to allow the organisation to achieve *both* one thing *and* the other. Moving from either/or polarities, dilemmas and tensions to both/and solutions is proving to be an essential shift in the cultural mind-set of all organisations that intend to survive and thrive through the ever-increasing paradoxes of the current working world (Cheal 2012).

## REFLECTION

Think of a recent change in your organisation. What sort of change was it? What evidence existed for the need for change? How effective was the change once implemented? What impacted on that degree of effectiveness?

# The Role of a Leader in Organisational Change

As a leader, you may find yourself in different roles (or a combination of roles) in connection with a change initiative:

- *Leading change*: This is where the change is initiated and driven by you and hence comes *from* you.

- *Managing change*: This is where the change is implemented by you and hence comes *through* you. This might be a change you yourself have initiated or, more usually, it is delegated from 'above', and you are required to 'make it happen' (whether you like it or not!). This would also include shared leadership structures where you are in the role of selling and communicating the change to others in the organisation.

- *Facilitating change*: This is where the change is supported by you and you are working *with* others to help them implement the change. This is the classic role of Organisational Development and HR consultants (in-house or external), where they are helping with the process but not necessarily delivering it themselves.

# The Context of a Change: The Big Picture

Every change will take place within a context or a 'frame'. At the start of any change initiative, it is important to establish the scope, for example:

- Who has initiated the change?
- Who are the stakeholders?

- Who is likely to be resistant and who is supportive?
- What are the boundaries?
- What is being delivered and what is *not* being delivered?
- What is changing and what is *not* changing?
- What is the change dependent on and what is dependent on it?
- What resources do you have?
- What restrictions are in place (e.g., policies, politics)?
- What are some of the forces for and against the change?

When considering the scope of the change within the organisation, a useful model to work with is the McKinsey 7S model (Peters and Waterman 1990). This model breaks an organisation down into seven components:

1. *Systems*: Including procedures, policies and IT systems

2. *Structure*: How the organisation is divided up, e.g., departments and levels

3. *Strategy*: Including plans, goals, targets and mission

4. *Shared values*: What is important to the organisation and the people, i.e., culture?

5. *Skills*: What does the organisation do? What skills do people have?

6. *Staff*: Who are the people? How many? How are they treated? Morale?

7. *Style*: The style of leadership and management, e.g., autocratic, supportive, etc.

The value of the model is in recognising that each of the components has a relationship with every one of the others. If you change one component, there will be a ripple effect through some of the others (and in this sense, the model is 'systemic'). For example, if you update Systems, you will also need to update the Skills, otherwise you will have demoralised Staff. (Systems thinking is covered in greater depth in Chapter 9.)

When initiating change, it is useful to establish:

- What specifically is changing in each of the components (*from* what *to* what)?
- How might each of the components impact on the change (positively and negatively)?
- How might the change impact on each of the components (positively and negatively)?

- What, if any, tensions exist between the components currently?
- What, if any, tensions might the change create between the components?

By understanding the 7Ss and exploring these questions, you are going to align your change with the way the organisation works. If your change is congruent with the 7Ss of the organisation, you have a greater chance of success.

## Using the 7S Model to Handle Uncertainty

In the health service industry of today, leaders have to get used to uncertainty, learning how to handle and embrace it. When layers of change are introduced into an already complex and dynamic environment (like the health service industry), the results can become genuinely unpredictable. Where chaos and uncertainty are a given, new initiatives can often bring about 'unintended consequences' (Merton 1996). It therefore benefits any leaders of change to familiarise themselves with the nature of systemic thinking (see Chapter 9).

For our purposes here, systemic thinking would mean understanding and exploring the potential 'ecology' (i.e., ripple effects) of a change to predict and hopefully prevent some of the otherwise unintended consequences. You can use the 7S model to consider the ecology of your change by asking for each of the Ss: 'What would happen if we did implement this change?' and 'What would happen if we didn't implement change?'

### REFLECTION

For a change you are planning in your organisation, use the 7S model and these two questions to explore your context in more depth. What new insight did this give you? What will you do differently as a result of that insight?

## The Psychology of Change: How to Gain Buy-In

In the same NHS report (Neath 2009, p. 4) mentioned previously, it was suggested that '70% of change programmes fail and 70% of those that fail do so because cultural barriers impede successful implementation.' The cultural barriers were measured by 'management behaviour not supportive of change' and 'employees resistant to change'.

In the initiation, planning and implementation phases of change, there is a need to build and maintain buy-in from various parties, particularly stakeholders, colleagues, management and staff. From observation, it is apparent that some leaders try to 'project manage' their way through change. Whilst project management is essential, it is usually not enough. The difference between change management and project management is the additional attention that needs to be given to people engagement. Linking back to the 7S model, there is a correlation between project management and the 'hard Ss' (systems, strategy and structure), and then between change management and the 'soft Ss' (shared values, staff, skills and style). Consider an office or department move. It is possible to treat the move as a project and manage it as such. However, if you don't take the feelings of the staff into account or involve them in the process, you may find yourself spending much of your time and budget handling disengaged staff, 'people issues' and increased staff turnover rather than managing the technicalities of the office move!

## Buy-In from Stakeholders and Collaborators

Stakeholders will tend to be those who could affect the change, those who are affected by the change or a combination of both. For any change you are leading, draw up a list of stakeholders (or stakeholder groups) and then ask yourself:

- How much power does each stakeholder have?
- How positive are they about the change?
- What is their intention in the change?

It is worth investing time in relationship building with anyone who has power over your change initiative in order to get them on board. These stakeholders are sometimes known affectionately as 'spanner-holders' because they have the potential to throw a spanner in the works! However, if they are engaged and bought in to your change, they also have the ability to help you by tightening or loosening things up.

One way to engage a stakeholder at the early stages is to ask what we call the 'involve' question. After pitching the need for the change, ask them for some input/advice, starting your request with something like: 'If you were involved in this change...' (e.g., 'If you were involved in this change... how would you X?' or '... who would be good to speak to about Y?' or '...what would we need to consider about Z?'). Not only is asking for their input/advice useful, but if they answer your question, they have also psychologically bought into the idea of the change. You can then utilise their suggestions (or the spirit of their suggestions) and let them know you have done this. Now, they know their idea has been incorporated and they are less likely to throw a spanner in the works. People don't tend to reject their own ideas!

Depending on who the stakeholder is, you may also need to 'contract' with them, i.e., set some basic agreements about roles and expectations. What do you need from them and what do they need from you? How will you communicate with them? How much collaboration and involvement do you want from them, and how much are they able to give?

The issue of contracting is also essential when working in collaboration with others. When setting up a collaborative-style partnership, we recommend you use the following as areas for agreement:

- What is the objective and purpose of the change? Is there a deadline?
- What is the ultimate deliverable of the change? How will things be different?
- What is negotiable and what is not?
- How will you know you have achieved the objective? How will others know? Is it measurable?
- What are the needs and desires of all parties? What would be considered a "win" for each party?
- How do you want to work together?
- How will you make decisions?
- How much time, budget and resources are available (or are parties willing to commit)?
- Are there any other expectations?
- What other outside influences could help/hinder the partnership/change?

Sometimes you will be working with people who want an alternative approach or outcome to that which you are proposing. If this is the case, seek to find out what it is they are attracted to and what the benefits are. By combining their benefits with the benefits of your own approach/ outcome, is there a 'third way' solution that meets the positives of both sides? By adopting a 'win/win' stance, you have a better chance of working through conflicting positions and turning a potential issue into an opportunity for a better solution.

## REFLECTION

Think of a change that was resisted. What was the intention of the stakeholders resisting the change? What change (if any) did they want to see and what 'third way' options might have been possible to offer a different route to getting needs met?

## Buy-In from Staff and Management

As well as stakeholders and collaborators, how do you encourage staff and management engagement? The simplest way to look at how human beings are influenced (e.g., to make a decision or to act in a certain way) is to imagine a seesaw in their mind(s). On one side of the seesaw is resistance and on the other side is motivation. If the collective resistance to change outweighs the motivation, then the change will be extremely challenging and time consuming. At worst it may not be sustained or it may even fail.

When considering resistance, some people might resist the content of the change (i.e., the 'what'), and some people might resist the process (i.e., the 'how'). Even if they do not resist the change itself, they may resist the feeling of *being changed*, particularly when they have a lack of input and perceived control. In addition, no matter how positive a change is, there is also likely to be some degree of loss. In this sense, resistance is often caused by the *fear of losing* something (e.g., security, control, status, knowledge, power, variety or working with people they like).

It is useful to draw up a list of what people's resistance might be to the change and then use that list as a basis to draw up a list of motivators for change. Remember, the motivators have to be applicable to them, not just to the organisation. For example, if the change means working in new teams and you have identified that a resistance might be working with people they don't know, make it clear that they will still be working with some of their current colleagues (if true) and that there will be some opportunities to meet and work (or socialise) with their new colleagues before the change takes place. Of course, it is important to avoid making promises that cannot be kept, as this will simply create another level of resistance.

In addition, you can help to counter the resistance by (a) removing some of it and (b) outweighing some of it with motivators. Ultimately, by acknowledging and understanding the resistance and using that to inform *how* you present, motivate and implement the change, you will tend to experience a smoother transition.

Some people don't see the need for change and are happy with the way things are now. In this instance, you may need to 'pace and lead' them. This means starting from their position and leading them to where you need to go. The first step is to create a sense of dissatisfaction with the current situation (e.g., start by talking about the current situation and what is not working). Then present the vision (i.e., the future outcome of how things could be along with the benefits of this outcome to the people and to the organisation). Finally, present the immediate tangible actions that will need to be taken to get the change underway. In addition, throughout this process, it is important to listen to concerns and to ensure support where possible.

As a final note on building and maintaining buy-in, it is essential that you manage both reality *and* perception. Not only do you need to deliver on the change project, you also need to keep people up to date with what you are delivering. If things change but people don't know or perceive that things have changed, they will continue to act as before, and systems are likely to return to the status quo! To prevent the change coming to a grinding halt, it is important to 'keep the wheels oiled' by consistently resolving resistance, inertia and practical issues in order to maintain momentum.

Your role, if you choose to accept it, is to lead yourself and your team within the institutional and professional context. Holding this multiple perspective is essential for successful implementation of any change.

## References

Cheal, J. 2012. *Solving impossible problems: Working through tensions and paradox in business.* Moggerhanger, GB: GWiz Publishing.

Merton, R. K. 1996. *On social structure and science.* Chicago: University of Chicago Press.

Neath, A. 2009. *Inspiring change in the NHS: Introducing the five frames.* NHS Institute for Innovation and Improvement. www.changemodel.nhs.uk/dl/cv_content/13772.

Peters, T., and R. Waterman. 1990. *In search of excellence: Lessons from America's best run companies.* New York: HarperCollins.

# 9 Second-Order Leadership

Mark Klaassen

## Introduction

Shakespeare once wrote a play entitled *Much Ado about Nothing* (1600).

There is also an old French proverb which says: 'The more things change, the more they remain the same'.

One of my clients—a frustrated leader in a community health organisation—turned red in the face as he expressed to me: 'I'm a known leader in this city, inspiring lots of progress activity, so how come *most of the change I want is NOT actually happening in my own organisation?*'

This represents a challenge often faced by leaders in the real world, whether in complex organisations, a department or a small business.

## Who Leads?

The word *leader* is a metaphor which presupposes *movement*. Leaders have followers, and they are following the lead—from somewhere to somewhere. Also presupposed in this metaphor of movement, is that some *change* is occurring—from some present state to a desired state; it's going somewhere, not staying in the same place. As such, leadership and change are intrinsically linked.

I think most leaders would agree that having a brilliant idea is less than half of what's needed to bring about significant change. Leading people through change effectively also requires more than the ability to have great vision and inspire people about it. Actually *getting the change to happen requires a clear awareness of **where** and **how** second-order change is required in the system.*

In the context of this book, these factors are true for a health organisation, a department or an individual healthcare professional.

Second-order change is what I will be talking about in this chapter. I am Mark Klaassen. As an internationally experienced NLP (Neuro-Linguistic Programming) master trainer, strategic facilitator and executive coach to a variety of large business and community organisations in New Zealand and Australia, I've had much opportunity to listen to leaders in some of their most difficult situations. While my primary field of application is business, I have over the years also worked with hospitals, medical school leadership and many doctors, and I earlier worked part-time in the psychiatric field for two years.

In previous chapters of this book, you may have read ideas and examples of what makes an effective practical leader, particularly in the context of a health organisation. In this chapter, I will outline:

- The differences between first- and second-order change
- The systemic thinking of a second-order leader
- The choice: second-order change or remaining at the effect of a dysfunctional system
- The question of more resources or differently organised resources
- The importance of using multiple-brain intelligences in healthcare practice
- The traps and illusions of thinking we have changed when we haven't

I also propose that to address the leadership frustration issues discussed previously, a second-order leader must *be a second-order thinker* and *use new language* for the second-order change desired.

This is much more than simply presenting a persuasive strategic theory of change.

## First- and Second-Order Change Theory

So let's begin with asking, 'What is the difference between first-order change and second-order change?'

*First-order change* is change that occurs within a system, which itself remains unchanged. The intention of first order change is to restore the existing system to functional fulfilment of its *original* purpose. You do first-order changes when the existing system has developed dysfunctions that prevent it from delivering the outputs for which it was originally designed.

First-order changes are like repairs to a car. They may be matters of maintenance or replacement of a faulty part with a fully functional part which is the same as the original. You still want this car to function in the same way it did when you bought it. Likewise, in an organisation, first-order changes are for the purpose of restoring the status quo and delivering the originally desired result.

First-order change looks at the past and asks the question 'why?' 'Why did this dysfunction happen, and how can we correct it?' This type of change has good purpose when the intention is to restore balance to the existing system and have it produce the results it used to deliver.

*Second-order change* is change from outside the system, which changes the system itself. It is generated by outside events or influences, and creates either a partially or fully new system, based on a different thought and paradigm, which will produce a different result than the original system.

Second-order change is driven by a perceived desirable future where different methods produce intentionally different results. It addresses the question 'how?' 'How can we get from now to the different desirable future?' It involves different thinking, different model/s, and different language to describe it, as it takes the players of such change into a different dimension.

First, let's look at a quick and simple example of second-order thinking.

## Example 9.1

Imagine a typical young family—mother, father and two children living in their own two-bedroom home. Mum and Dad have one bedroom and the children share the other. A few years later when they have a third baby, and that child grows old enough to need a full-sized bed, they have a problem: There is no room to put another bed in the existing bedrooms, no other significant space in the home, and no room to add another bed into the floor space of the children's bedroom.

First-order change would simply be to try reshuffling all sorts of furniture in order to make a third bed fit. This will not achieve a satisfactory result, and is much like a lot of the restructuring which organisations put themselves through at the effect of first-order thinking. It's like re-arranging the deck chairs on the *Titanic*, still heading to an iceberg.

Consider the possibility of second-order change. What do *you* think the options are for this family? Second-order change requires thinking outside the box, in another dimension. For example, they could bring in bunkbeds— adding a bed in an upward dimension not requiring extra floor space. Or they could add another room onto their house, which may require some temporary disruption but would achieve the desired result and add value to the home.

And now let's consider a hospital-based example.

## Example 9.2

An A&E clinic is having significant complaints due to errors in patient treatment. When challenged why this continues, the head of department says, 'We need more staff'. After some discussions in various meetings, more money is provided for more staff and they get more staff. However, nearly a year later, complaints are still flowing in much the same nature and quantity.

So what to do? Unhappy with the idea of just shelling out more money, the hospital administrators bring in a consultant with a background in systems thinking and organisational flow. The consultant spends about three weeks doing research into the real causes of the complaints and errors, and comes back with a report saying the issue was not caused by the number of staff; the problems actually lie in the areas of communication and process.

> In particular, within the culture of the department, the poor communication and relationship skills of some leaders were resulting in many staff simply doing what they were told, and not feeling able to challenge or question the decisions.

> Also, some processes and procedures within the department were dysfunctional, and resulted in things like: information not being passed on to where it was needed in time, some staff not having information access or authority they needed, and a notable lack of checking the assessments and key decisions about patient health and treatment, plus a lack of consistent follow-up to ensure action had been implemented.

Of course the department leaders challenged the consultant's view as being isolated and generally not true, but the consultant had a variety of case studies illustrating the facts, showing the problem to be endemic throughout the department.

So after months of arguing, the hospital administrators finally appointed the consultant as project manager to a small team for evaluating and implementing changes to address the issues as outlined. This also resulted in two changes in leadership staff.

> A further evaluation three months after the implementation of these changes showed significant shifts in the communication culture, increased acceptance of responsibility, reduction of errors and thus of complaints, and a gradual—although not universal—willingness to cooperate between layers of the team.

> It was further noted that this type of change required significant discussion with, and persuasion of, medical leaders—some of whom were not initially willing participants in the change. As hospital culture is commonly hierarchical, general staff needed to be acquainted with better ways to ask questions or even challenge a decision without being disrespectful of the team leader or doctor. Also, in this culture, those with power were reluctant at first to change to a more egalitarian

rather than dictatorial communication style. The realizations came gradually that:

- Relating in mutual respect created better communication solutions than issuing orders.
- Staff acting from fear of reprisal reduced the clarity, efficiency and quality of work.
- Perhaps the hierarchical model of medical teams is not the best option anymore.

More often than not, the flurry of activity that occurs in organisations, with the intention of creating new change and new results, does not produce the desired results because their leaders are unaware that they are reshuffling the first-order system, *not* creating a second-order system.

A *different* result may truly be required, and even though they talk about working smarter and working harder, nothing really significant changes, and more of the same is produced (Ashby, 1956).*

In the hospital example presented here, more staff just became more people reinforcing the same system dysfunctions. A different system was required to bring second-order change and the desired result.

There is a biblical parable of the wineskins (Luke 5:37) in which Jesus says:

> And no man puts new wine into old bottles; else the new wine will burst the bottles, and be spilled, and the bottles shall perish. But new wine must be put into new bottles; and then both are preserved.

One of the points being made here is that the fermentation process of new wine and the wineskins makes the wineskins brittle by the time the wine is ready to drink. Sometimes to shortcut the process, people would try putting new wine in the old wineskins; then the new fermentation process would crack the old wineskins, so you lose both the wine and the wineskins.

Like in the parable of the wineskins, trying to get a second-order result by forcing change on a first-order non-change system will often break the first-order system apart and cause greater problems and disruption, without producing the desired result.

## When You Need to Challenge Current Thinking

*Some* types of change—in an organisation, or department or even a person—require a brand new system or strategy to be installed. For example,

---

* Paraphrased here is Ross Ashby's Law of Requisite Variety, which says: 'Resilience, adaptability and determination are essential qualities for change leaders in a large organisation, because the masses often show considerable adaptability in returning cultural change processes to the status quo'.

- In some systems, there is too much resistance built in for the desired change to be adopted, so it will do its best to revert. This resistance may be in processes or may come through people.

- In some cases, too much disruption would be caused by the change to the existing system.

In these cases, a common solution approach is to allow the dysfunctional system to continue to operate and provide the current level of service, while a new second-order system is built, trialed and proven to deliver the new desired output. When it is ready, the second-order system will take over, and the original system will be disengaged.

Note that system replacement is only required in *some* sorts of second-order change.

## Choose to Change or to Be at Effect of Change?

George Land (1973) (author, innovator and systems scientist) says, contrary to the common adage:

> If you do the same old thing in the same old way, eventually you will *not* get the same old result.

'Why?' you might ask. Well think about how this is true in business.

For example, a large stationery business was successful for many years by doing things the way it did. And then suddenly they found they were losing market share, and the business owners wondered 'why?' After talking with their staff, they put new paint and signage on the front of the shop and put out a new glossy brochure. These changes made little impact on the business. In actual fact, the loss of market share was because consumer needs had changed, and their competitors were providing better service and better pricing. So continuing to use the same system and spending marketing dollars on it was not going to improve their result in a significant way. The owners had to change significantly in those three areas, or their business would have become insolvent.

Likewise, in a relationship between two people, certain behaviours by one person may be tolerated for a certain amount of time, but then the other person hits a threshold on his or her tolerance and will no longer put up with the same old behaviours. Whereas before, when apologies and minor behavioural adjustments were permitted, now the game has changed, and a major shift is required. Either shift to an entirely different range of behaviours that get the desired result, or go find another relationship!

One of the key points here is that if we, as healthcare leaders, do not *choose* the second-order change that would produce the desired results (even if that involves some pain), then inevitable change will be forced upon us by the levels of dysfunction and poor results in the existing system.

In these days, when health systems around the world are most commonly underfunded, there is often resistance to making more than cosmetic changes. However, when viewed on a macro scale over a period of years, less money and resources would be wasted by making a powerful second-order change sooner while also achieving the desired results in a much shorter time frame.

## Do We Need More Resources, or Reorganised Resources?

When resources are limited, change can sometimes be achieved within our current circumstances by second-order thinking. The secret here is to retain the organisational content with key knowledge and skills, and then to reorganise your resources in a manner that will increase performance *and* take out the resistance that prevents change.

In the classic movie *Ben-Hur* (1959), there is a chariot race which Ben-Hur must win. He is up against a strong opponent who has superior horses. So what should he do, how could he win? As the story goes, he met an old wise horseman, who pointed out that Ben-Hur had horses of different styles and speed on his team—they were good horses, but not getting top performance. The old man advised Ben-Hur: 'Since the race is a large circle around the Coliseum, I suggest you put your slow and steady horse on the inside of the racing circle, and the high-flying fast horse on the outside!' He won!

Do you notice how he achieved that? The same horses, in the same situation—organised a different way—produced a superior result.

Clockmakers who make the old grandfather clocks understand clockworks. One thing they know is that there are some cogs on a big old grandfather clock which you could hold in vain and not actually stop the clock. There are one or two other cogs, usually small ones, on which a simple touch would stop the whole clock mechanism. The key, of course, is knowing where to touch and how.

As a healthcare leader, restructuring of teams or organisational change will only get the best results when using second-order systemic thinking.

# Beware of Cyclical Sameness

There is a model of change based around the sigmoid curve (George Land again) which says that change goes through three phases:

- *Formative*: where there is a new beginning based on an idea, which begins to be introduced.

- *Normative*: where the new ways become common practice, the norm.

- *Integrative*: a phase where the normative way is reaching its peak, and for various reasons also needs to prepare for a new phase of change or it risks decline. Hence integrating the current system into the next new phase of change is required. This latter is called developmental change.

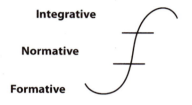

**Integrative**

**Normative**

**Formative**

Second-order change produces developmental change, which in the sigmoid curve model would look like the progressive upward growth sequence of developmental change figure below—one phase feeding into the next level.

**Developmental Change**                    **Cyclical Sameness**

However, the illusion of organisational leaders is often more like that of cyclical sameness figure, above. This illustrates that even though some activity and so-called restructuring is occurring, essentially the same results are being produced because the system remains much the same. First-order changes—simply rearranging—do not result in second-order outcomes.

By way of illustration, it's like a woman who had trouble sustaining a long-term relationship. She kept complaining to her friends that she had no trouble starting a relationship, but could not keep it going. She was overheard to say to one friend, 'I changed my style of clothing and I dyed my hair red, but still the relationship didn't last'... and to another friend a few months and another relationship later: 'This time I was going out with a sailor, not a mechanic like the last two times, but we still broke up after four months'. Obvious as it may seem to many, she was missing the main point—that the changes she was making were cosmetic rearrangements, but she had not changed her ways of relating in a relationship.

A key point here is that second-order change can never be cyclical sameness; it must always be developmental change. This will include a change of the paradigm agreements which guide how we function and communicate together in order to achieve a significantly different result. Otherwise, you get to relive the phrase: 'The more things change, the more things remain the same'.

I recently heard of an example of second-order change among radiographers. In order to reduce the need for doctors to be involved in every decision arising from a scan or X-ray, assessments were done and it was recognised that some radiographers have the experience and knowledge to make mid-level decisions around patient care. So radiography has been evaluated and categorised into four levels (from assistant to consultant practice, as outlined in Chapter 7), with variant operational functions and authority, according to their knowledge and skill. This alleviated the need for doctors to attend to so many matters, reduced waiting times for patients, increased the job satisfaction of advanced radiographers, and gave junior radiographers something more to aspire to.

Another example being adopted in some hospitals involves a more holistic approach to wellness, where a person in the hospital after a heart attack is not just a 'heart patient'. Instead, the patient is recognized as a person with a life, work, dietary patterns, relationships, and other habits and events—all of which are now taken into account and explored with regard to the treatment plan, which is co-created with the patient.

I am often asked the question: 'Why don't we have more second-order thinkers in our organisations?' My observation is that there are always second-order thinkers in an organisation; however, there is a ratio effect: The more hierarchical dominance that exists in a culture, the less permission and funding there is for second-order thinkers to express their outside-the-box thinking, challenging the existing culture and taking action to generate trial models of operation. So the answer is that we do not have a culture that allows and supports second-order thinking.

## Multiple Brain Leadership

A new field in leadership development technology is mBIT (Multiple Brain Integration Techniques), which has a powerful effect on self-leadership and complex decision making. This is perhaps one of the most progressive second-order breakthroughs in personal and professional development in the last decade. (The topic is referred to again in Chapter 16.)

The scientific fact that both the heart and the enteric gut are each actually a brain, carrying out major neural network functions both alone and in conjunction with the head brain, means that better communications and results can now be gained for:

- The self (decision making on neural awareness of relevant feedback previously disregarded)
- The patient (checking/responding what their cardiac and enteric brains are telling them)
- Communication between staff about multiple brain insights, creating superior quality and more holistic treatment options for a patient and changing the way we do leadership in health care

More than 600 papers have been written which relate to this field, and the results support the notion that mental thought and allopathic medicine are not the only significant contributors to applications of wellness.

## Leading in Complex Systems

In the complex system that is an organisation, filled with many people, many roles and many agendas, *key leaders* need to have a *point of difference*. If these leaders are to be effective and second-order level, that point of difference will essentially be how they think and whether they use a different set of language patterns that clearly articulate how the second-order model differs from the first.

Complex organisations have a range of stakeholders, each frequently espousing different outcomes and offering opposing arguments with regard to how something should be done, who should get the most resources and what the priorities ought to be. What helps is that the other leaders generally carry a common identity as people working together in the service of an organisation and its outcomes. The leverage this gives to key leaders is that they can link their language to the higher level of organisational outcomes and seek to draw the various departmental and individual outcomes into alignment, based around:

- How well each leader contributes to the achievement of organisational outcomes
- How well they *interface with other departments* and processes in doing so

Often, too much attention is paid to *what* we will change and not enough is paid to *how* we will make those changes. Especially important in any change process is the quality of interface between systems and the communication example set by key leaders.

Another short-term option that second-order leaders will frequently use to evaluate effectiveness—guiding whether we make a particular change or not

**Table 9.1:** Cartesian Questions Chart

| X, Y | X, –Y |
|---|---|
| What will happen if you do … ? | What will happen if you don't … ? |
| –X, Y | –X, –Y |
| What won't happen if you do … ? | What won't happen if you don't … ? |

and also how best to bring about that change—is a tool like the Cartesian questions (Table 9.1). Having a board, committee or group evaluate an issue based on these questions helps people see things from a systemic point of view. Also useful are *causal loops diagrams* (Google this term for more information).

Sometimes even a plan with a second-order intention does not work because it has not been given sufficient systemic thought, i.e., about how the change will affect other aspects of the system beyond those intended to be changed. Sometimes such matters are recognised, but some are swept under the carpet.

Here are some examples of issues in healthcare organisations when it is useful to have facilitated systemic discussions toward second-order change in today's demanding environment:

- Deciding whether we spend the money on these resources or those resources, when we can't buy all the resources that would be desired.

- Choosing a course when doctors are having some of their roles undertaken by other disciplines, like nurses, radiographers and midwives. More important than just considering the advantages and disadvantages is working through the wider implications of such changes, how to interface the new roles well, and checking whether indeed this is second-order change or simply a tweak to the existing system.

If a second-order thinker/facilitator does not exist within the organisation, it may be appropriate to bring in an external consultant, whose expertise may in the end save time and money in change effectiveness.

# Make Use of Chaos

Leaders in complex systems will often experience chaos. The good news is that this chaos can be used to your advantage. Looking at systems in the light of Ilya Prigogine's book, *Order Out of Chaos* (1984), he points out that a big stress on a system seeks a new flow direction. For example, a logjammed river seeks another route for the water to flow; commuters at a standstill every day in peak-hour traffic seek another way to travel or different hours of work. The point is that sometimes there needs to be enough pressure or pain to create the change, and in these times, strong articulate second-order leadership stands out with superior results.

## In Conclusion

To create second-order change, often an external consultant is required in the short term. In due course, the ideal is for second-order leaders to be trained and developed within the organisation. This is where NLP comes into its own, in alignment with systems thinking and the new field of mBIT (Multiple Brain Integration Techniques) (Oka and Soosalu, 2012).

## References

Ashby, Ross. *An Introduction to Cybernetics*. London: Chapman and Hall, 1956.

Ben-Hur. (1959). William Wyler, director. Hollywood, CA: Metro-Goldwyn-Mayer.

Land, George. *Grow or Die: The Unifying Principle of Transformation.* New York: Random House, 1973.

Oka, Marvin and Grant Soosalu. *mBraining: Using Your Multiple Brains to Do Cool Stuff* (2012). www.mBraining.com.

Prigogine, Ilya and Isabelle Stengers. *Order Out of Chaos: The Evolutionary Paradigm and the Physical Sciences* (1984), New York: Bantam, 290 pp.

# 10 Inspiring Others to Follow Your Lead: Leading Change

Anna McNaughton and David Collier

This chapter leads on from the concept of institutional change to looking at how you inspire others to follow you in the change you want to see in your workplace and your wider profession. Two elements of this chapter stand side by side and beg the question: 'Are all inspiring leaders people who bring about change?' Looking dispassionately at this, it seems prudent to initially break the two elements apart and consider first what an inspiring leader is, and then consider how change might be led. Then perhaps we might consider the relationship between inspirational leadership and change.

## REFLECTION

- What is inspirational leadership?
- Who and where have you seen it in your workplace or life?

## Inspirational Leadership

Inspirational leadership is often a challenge, especially in large, complex organisations with well-entrenched professional cultures and traditions. This is the situation in the healthcare world.

A sound and useful starting point from which to begin this discussion is to look at this concept of leadership specifically in light of the many leaders we see daily through the prism of our media. Our understanding of their work is limited to the brief comments made to capture attention and support the requisite agenda of the person and the day. There is little evidence given of considered and thoughtful opinion or of the decision making underpinning these leaders' actions. What appears to matter is that the 'leader' is seen to be doing something, to be behaving as a LEADER should. The outcome of this 'action-driven leadership' is that the general population no longer understands what leadership is. One of the early examples of this apparent interference from the top, seizing-the-headlines approach must be that of Winston Churchill on January 3, 1911, when he personally attended the siege of Sidney Street. He wrote at the time that whatever his other motives, 'I must, however, admit that convictions of duty were supported by a strong sense of curiosity which perhaps it would have been well to keep in check' (Smith n.d.).* It is worth noting to Churchill's credit that his only interference was to suggest that the containment lines be extended while refusing to allow the fire brigade to approach the fire that engulfed the house. So this example clarifies the things that leadership is not.

## Modern Healthcare Environments

We live and work in a world where there are now many safety considerations which are part of everyday healthcare business—considerations that some see as barriers to leadership. It is not uncommon to hear people admiring those individuals such as Jeremy Clarkson from the BBC TV show *Top Gear* for his uncompromising attitudes towards most forms of political correctness. In a marketing sense for that programme, it is highly effective; as a tool to appeal to everyone's frustration with endless rules and officious bureaucracy, it is also highly effective; and as a source of humorous connection to the audience, it is ideal. However, would you want to have him as a leader? He does not pretend to be that, nor does he advocate widely his style in fronting the *Top Gear* team, and in all truthfulness, he evokes responses from the public which encompass the complete spectrum of possible opinion towards him. This highlights the difference between recognition and leadership, and it is important that this distinction be kept in mind. It would seem that many modern politicians seek, not unreasonably, to ensure that they are recognised, and it is we who make the mistake of assuming that leadership and recognition are one and the same thing. This distinction is a key point and one which we hope might make you stop and think about leadership in a revised light. It should also lead you to consider that different environments, such as health care, as distinct from entertainment or business, require different attributes for their leaders.

---

* This example is provided explicitly to identify one of the better early examples of a politician using an event to strengthen his or her public profile and yet also acknowledge that such action was 'inappropriate'.

## REFLECTION

- Do you agree or disagree with this? (Do we need a different sort of leader in health care?)
- In your opinion, what are the different attributes required of healthcare leaders in your organisation?
- Do you have these attributes?

# Forms of Inspiration

Roland Huntford (1979/1999), in his comparative biography of Amundsen and Scott's race to be first to the South Pole, was scathing in his assessment of Scott as a leader. In contrast, he highlighted the polar credentials and organisation of Amundsen, which led to the Norwegian success, as distinct from the preparations and planning which made up the Scott expedition. It is a book worth reading if only on the level of building an awareness of how the leader's role can play out in practice. These two individuals do provide a sound starting point in this present discussion, as they highlight the meaning of inspiration. Huntford is convincing in demonstrating the methodical and thoughtful preparation provided by both men in mounting their expeditions to the South Pole. From this, it can be noted that both planned their journeys based on their knowledge and experience, and this is all too frequently the source of leadership failure, where the knowledge and experience used by the leaders is not appropriate, or current, for the situation in which it is required. We all use knowledge and experience to form our thoughts; the question is how to recognise when that is insufficient for the place or the person to be able to rely upon it. It is at this point that inspirational leaders are able to call on their sub-leaders and wider team to question and challenge the plan before it is put into practice. From reading on these two men, Scott and Amundsen, it is evident that there was discussion and agreement, but it is unclear as to whether there was questioning about the organisational structure that had been put together until they were in place at the Antarctic and therefore unable to make radical adjustments to their plans. It is not the place of this chapter to explore leadership failure, but clearly this line of thinking should encourage you to reflect upon this aspect of leadership.

Both Amundsen and Scott evoked a very strong degree of loyalty and faith from those they were leading. Was that loyalty from organisational necessity? Scott was a senior naval officer, and his team was largely drawn from the military, where, in those times, obedience was of paramount importance. Was it from environmental location and the isolation of the Antarctic, with its interrelated imperative that in that environment, and for everyone's survival, they must be able to rely completely on each other? Or was it that Scott and Amundsen were inspirational leaders? There is evidence that both teams found their leader 'inspirational', credible, someone whom they wished to follow, but did they inspire their teams to believe in themselves? This is the crux of inspiring others to follow: that individuals should be able to follow even in the leader's absence.

## A DEFINITION OF AN INSPIRATIONAL LEADER

The definition of an inspirational leader can be someone who inspires you, the follower, to believe in yourself. To do that effectively, you need to both know yourself and you need leaders who not only know themselves, but also acknowledge their strengths and weaknesses openly.

This definition, in its scope, would remove all of those individuals mentioned previously from consideration. It would exclude seemingly most present-day political leaders, though some, such as Nelson Mandela, would have comfortably fit into such a description, but he was clearly a man of unusual and enviable moral depth and strength. The manner in which this definition lends itself best to our use is in that of causing us to focus on the purpose of leadership. Is leadership something for the benefit of the person aspiring to be the leader, or is it for the purpose of benefitting the organisation and even mankind? To put it more plainly, is leadership egocentric or is it altruistic?

One might argue then that an inspirational leader is one who has the benefit of mankind as the prime purpose, but there's the rub. What one person might see as a benefit to mankind may and in fact will not be shared by everyone. So there needs to be further conversation and clarity around this definition. It will not be adequate to look at different types of leaders for an answer because, although they may give us case-by-case insight, these cases will not in the end answer the subjective issue of what is best for mankind. So can we argue that an inspirational leader might be seen as one who leads for the benefit of mankind? One would not think so; this cannot be their core motivation, nor should we accept that this defines an 'inspirational leader'. There are always examples of some of the more repugnant leaders in our history who were frequently described by their supporters in glowing terms—words like *messianic*, *inspirational* and *glorious* are commonplace for such people.

A solution emerges when looking at past dictatorial leaders, and it is found in their common failing to care for anyone other than themselves. They see themselves as the centre of the universe, as superior beings who are justified in living according to their own rules. There is a psychological term for this sort of behaviour, and it is not uncommon in business leadership to encounter people who display these traits, often charming and witty, great company and exciting to be with, for a while. Their values and their sense of responsibility for their actions are, however, non-existent. What we should be looking for is a leader providing a genuine commitment to other peoples' well-being and that leader building those peoples' belief in themselves. The moral imperative is about moral depth and strength and integrity. Inspirational leaders don't just talk the talk, they walk the walk and they very likely do not think of themselves as either egocentric or altruistic. They are focussed on providing this genuine commitment to their task. It is as a consequence of this focus that, in leading change, they also lead belief in that change so that their followers can easily have a commitment to it. It is part of their belief in themselves.

An inspirational leader then is someone who is strongly altruistic and who leads you, the follower, to believe in yourself.

This opening attempt to define the type of leader who might inspire others to follow their lead sets the scene for this chapter. We propose now to look closely at the qualities and behaviours which appear to us to be necessary for a genuinely inspirational leader and in the process explore the place of such leaders in leading change.

## What Makes an Inspirational Leader?

There is a wide range of views about what makes up the various essentials for inspirational leadership, and motivational speakers around the world present various theories on this topic. In essence, it would seem that there are just a few common and key components which drive those theories.

1. Enthusiasm

2. Communication

3. Belief in the direction and the team

The hardest to maintain is enthusiasm, and in our view, the most difficult to ensure is communication. Many moments in our current working lives are spent preparing for meetings and delivering goals and objectives to the work teams. It is a commonplace criticism that organisations do not honour their commitments in these regards or do so in a perfunctory fashion. A good example which many of us may have encountered are those meetings where we have gathered to hear options and discuss the direction and plan only to find that in fact the exercise is one of rubber-stamping a pre-arranged outcome. A modern variation is the call for submissions with impossibly tight deadlines so that few are able to genuinely canvas opinion. The impact of this casual and cursory approach and attitude on follower enthusiasm is dramatic. It has an emotional impact on individuals, and as Carlson states in *Psychology: The Science of Behaviour*, 'Emotions are intimately related to motivation' (1984, p. 523). Clearly then, this is a challenge for anyone leading a team, to bring a freshness and enthusiasm to their role and their direction that they are trying to lead their team towards, which will then motivate their followers to feel inspired.

It is worrying that so many people we speak with seem to feel that their attendance at work is simply functional, and that no matter what an individual might do, those higher up the leadership chart do not recognise the value of those they are leading. In part this comes about due to external forces, of which failure to pay salaries on time is the most critical. However, for those in the health sector who have taken up their roles with the aspiration of 'helping others', the very structures within which they work come to be seen as obstructive, blocking initiative and supporting the frequent opinion that they are favouring those who play the game better.

This leads to the question, 'What lies behind this viewpoint?' How can we explain and understand this opinion, and most importantly, how can we address and resolve the issue? Inspiring others to follow your lead can be a challenging option at times, especially when some statistics suggest that many, perhaps the majority of people are ambivalent, and in our view as many as 20% may actually be disengaged. We all know about the Pareto principle, which will see us concentrating 80% of our time on this 20%. This tends to draw the leaders back into detailed management, facing the challenge of trying to engage and inspire them or actually keep them from stuffing up. This mind-set and how we engage is often the difference between management and leadership.

Many people write off disengaged staff rather than trying to engage and understand the issues and how the person feels which leads them to believe that they cannot connect to the organisation's values or plans. Often it is a result of being let down or frustrated by promises or changes from the organisation. This group of people can be your biggest threat to performance or could be your greatest opportunity if you aim to work with them rather than against them.

It was suggested by Zenger and Folkman (2013) that when leaders were more proactive in reaching out—looking for issues, trends, opportunities and potential problems which then assisted others to support and embrace the change and encouraged others to do so—then that positive action produced more successful leaders.

## Inspirational Change

So change, and inspirational change at that, is the answer. These attitudes are indicators that change is necessary, and sooner rather than later. Looking back to our definition of an inspirational leader, it is clear that they must be able to inspire their followers to believe in themselves. A simple task to achieve this is to get feedback from followers, either formally or informally, but the essential task is to find out what they think, where they think they are going and what ideas they might have to help us all to get there. This needs to be done with a genuine interest to hear and understand their perspectives. Take the time to fully analyse the constructive feedback both positive and critical and internalise these so as to produce a response in which people can recognise their own ideas playing an integral part, properly acknowledged, in the overall direction of the team and the overall delivery of health services. This depth of participation creates ownership and self-belief that each person is valued because their contribution is part of the plan. It goes to the heart of building a positive and supportive culture within an organisation.

This plan is a plan for change, and now the leader must keep the motivation by bringing it about in a way which is well communicated. Garbled or mixed messages are a regularly reported management issue in our surveying of membership (Castletine-Jackson and Mercer 2012). This happens in the average workplace on a daily basis, and therefore it is incumbent on an inspirational leader to send very clear messages repeatedly and regularly. Have your team looking out for the update or the reinforcement of the original message. All of us get very busy and have fallen into the trap of thinking, 'Oh well, nothing is changing this week, so I have nothing to say'. The very absence of a message is, in itself, saying something and, worse, it is saying something that other people will interpret. Imagine for a moment how uncontrollable that piece of information will be.

Our second key component, then, is to have effective communication strategies that are constantly assessed and reviewed. Everyone must be part of this and be encouraged to take up the fundamentals of good communication and asking questions too. (Maybe take the time to revisit Chapter 4 and reflect again on your communication skills.) This is a key part of a leader's own learning. The leader inspiring change should constantly encourage the asking of questions. What most leaders find most frustrating about questions is when they are asked questions that have obvious answers or are completely unrelated to the direction of the communication. Both of these tend to suggest that the questioner has not been paying attention or has not prepared for the moment. A good leader often reflects and asks the question, 'So why does this person not have the story yet?' Or, 'What has to be true for this person to be seeing this situation as they do?' Another way in which to address this is to ask staff to come prepared to ask questions having reflected on the situation. What should be gained from asking questions is clarity and understanding, and if we do this as part of the team, then everyone gains a better insight. It is even more satisfying when some glorious person asks a question that has not been considered, and this opens up even more exciting directions and opportunities for the team. Once staff are encouraged and supported to ask questions, you will find they will do so with enthusiasm and intense excitement, which they carry over into the world around them because it too has become an exciting place in which to question what is.

Bringing this practice into the workplace may initially be frustrating, since so many of our fellow workers appear to have lost the fun of questioning, perhaps being too busy 'doing stuff', fearful of the response questions might get, or the sense that looking like you don't have the answers may be a career-limiting view. Work environments may tend to be serious, but that doesn't mean that you have to be stiff all the time. One of the best opportunities to inspire your team to follow your lead is to be animated. Body language plays a significant role in communication and can be an asset or a challenge working in multi-ethnic health organisations.

Using our body language, including facial expressions and gestures, is one of the most effective communication strategies we can adopt in the workplace. Most people have to do presentations at some point in their careers. The stiff leader behind the lectern hardly motivates those in attendance, whereas the energetic, engaged and passionate leader who connects, who often moves around and talks to the individuals in the room, engaging easily with an engaging smile and the use of eye contact, demonstrates a real presence. We are used to performance, to presenters acting, so it is incumbent upon leaders to be prepared to be larger than life in their communication style—without being insincere or over the top.

If we are trying to inspire change, such an approach is vital. Inspirational leaders communicate *with* their audience as part of the team, not to them. Some of the greatest leaders in speaking would digress into stories on the side, whimsical and amusing but always with a point. There are a range of other practical actions that can be easily taken to inspire people to lead, such as looking at role models and their behaviours, their skills and attitudes, which is why we started this chapter with some historical examples.

## REFLECTION

- When you think about being inspired to change, who or what is the first thought that pops into your head?
- What are the actions that they do? What/who has inspired you in the past?
- What don't they do? What actions detract from any positive future direction?
- What can you learn from this about things to start AND to stop doing in being a leader that inspires change?

Peter Drucker spoke about how 'we spend a lot of time helping leaders learn what to do.... We don't spend enough time helping leaders learn what to stop doing' (Goldsmith and Reiter 2007, p. 35). This takes us onto the subject of role modelling and walking the talk. Our final overriding obligation is to take accountability for your actions as a leader even when things go wrong, and even when it was someone else's direct responsibility (whilst always acknowledging positive results to those in the team responsible and not taking the credit for yourself).

## Being an Inspirational Role Model

One of the complaints frequently heard about leadership in the healthcare environment is the habit of individuals and groups passing the blame upwards without acknowledging their own accountability. It can commonly be expressed in the phrase 'Why do we have to do this if senior management are not?' So often people lead in a 'do what I say, not what I do' manner. It should not be surprising, then, that their teams remain disengaged, confused or even defiant. They become leaders without followers and leaders without support.

Every leader who aspires to empowering their team, who wants to encourage their team to believe in themselves, has at some time acknowledged something along the lines of the following statement from a client who said:

> One of my greatest manager/leader/coach moments was when I was wrong.... People can learn so much from mistakes. I had stuffed up and I admitted it publically in front of my team. The other important part was taking responsibility to fix it and fixing it. In being upfront about it, saying how I was going to fix it and getting support about this, allowed my new team to see that it was OK to make mistakes and that taking responsibility was a better way of working than hiding it or making excuses. It provided a greater openness in the workplace, where staff could see I was human and made mistakes AND I was also a leader who took ownership, accountability and responsibility for my behaviour and actions.

There are many versions of the 'above the line and below the line' model. (See previous comments on 'cause and effect' in Chapters 3 and 4.) However, it remains one of the simplest yet most effective models to engage leaders in communication, leadership style and morale of team.

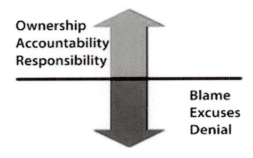

Recognising and responding actively with all of these tools effectively will almost certainly inspire a belief in both the direction and the team. It is this belief which is going to bring about a solid support for your leadership and the implementation of the change which is planned or about to be undertaken.

## References

Carlson, N. R. 1984. *Psychology: The science of behaviour*. Boston: Allyn and Bacon.

Castletine-Jackson, J., and N. Mercer. 2012. *BIR survey of AIR membership, 2011*. British Institute of Radiology.

Goldsmith, M., and M. Reiter. 2007. *What got you here won't get you there: How successful people become even more successful*. New York: Hyperion.

Huntford, R. 1979/1999. *Scott and Amundsen*. New York: Random House.

Smith, S. n.d. *The siege of Sidney Street*. Churchill Centre and Museum. http://www.winstonchurchill.org/learn/biography/radical/the-siege-of-sidney-street.

Zenger, J., and J. Folkman. 2013. *How poor leaders become good leaders*. HBR Blog Network. http://blogs.hbr.org/cs/2013/02/how_poor_leaders_become_good_l.html.

# 11 Motivating and Engaging Others: Driving Practice Change

Bev Snaith and Maryann Hardy

If you ask people how they have changed practice, they would probably find it difficult to answer in a single sentence, as it often relates so intangibly to situation, personal experience and the individuals around them. This chapter takes a more detailed look at how to lead change in health care, particularly in the context of practice, professional or role boundaries.

## Introduction

The word *leader* is one which evokes many different reactions within individuals, commonly based on experience, whether related to a personal encounter or media propaganda. Similarly, a seemingly infinite number of definitions of the term *leadership* exist. Northouse (2007, p. 3) describes it as 'a process whereby an individual influences a group of individuals to achieve a common goal'; whereas Knippenberg and Hogg (2004, p. 6) suggest it is 'a process of social influence in which the leader enlists the talents and efforts of others to accomplish the chosen task'. Denning (2007, p. 217) describes it as 'the ability to connect people to meaningful goals without hierarchical power to compel compliance'. However, all these definitions relate to the characteristics of an individual and their ability to work with, and influence, those around them. But healthcare leaders may work within a single, or multiple, team(s) each comprising individuals (practitioners, patients and/or carers) with their own beliefs and skills coming together with a single purpose to deliver high-quality care.

Internationally, clinical practice is continually evolving, facilitated by technological advances, research evidence and collaboration, but it is also driven by the increasing knowledge and expectations of patients, carers and practitioners. No matter where in the world health care is delivered, change is inevitable. National policies will continue to drive local innovation, whether to improve outcomes, service access and efficiency, or to save money. The key challenge in implementing changes in practice is to engage a (potentially diverse) group of individuals and engender a common purpose (Kings Fund 2012) and innovations may fail due to a lack of understanding of the potential impact of developments on other people or systems.

This chapter aims to assist the reader to develop an understanding of the challenges and opportunities of engaging those around them to implement changes in practice. Whether in a permanent role involving leadership of clinicians or practice, or as a 'change agent' managing a specific project impacting on health professionals, the principles are the same; however, actions may vary depending on relationships (short or long term), knowledge and experience.

## Planning Change

Often perceived small-scale changes such as the recruitment of a new team member, or engaging a different equipment supplier, can be as disruptive and challenging as a move to a new facility. Change calls for planning and coordination, skills that not every leader possesses, but which will be valuable in effectively improving practice.

Do not rush in; as a leader it is important not to jump straight to implementation and examining resourcing implications. Once the vision is established then plans to implement the service changes need to be drawn up and agreed by the relevant decision-making bodies. This is normally a high-level process to agree on the next steps and identify timescales and team members. The risk at this stage is that you try and implement change with the current resources and services and decide it is not possible, rather than considering all the alternatives.

### CASE STUDY

### Using Critical Incident Analysis

In an attempt to re-organise patient pathways and provide a new musculoskeletal service in the community, James was tasked with drawing up the plans. He could not see how it would work with the current number of specialist doctors and therapists, and he wanted to plan for recruitment and expansion. However, as there was not yet organisational buy-in for the service, a paper was required for the strategic planning committee. Four weeks later, no paper was forthcoming, and eventually another manager was asked to take on the project.

## REFLECTION

James was unable to draw up a high-level plan and could only think about the impact on him and his staff.

- What could he have done differently?
- Have you seen others do something similar?
- Can you step back and look at the big picture? What different opinions and options open up in doing this?

# Sharing the Vision of Change

You may be asked (or have personally identified an opportunity) to make changes in practice by reviewing a patient pathway, introducing cross-boundary working, or implementing evidence-based research outcomes. Whatever the justification, it is important that the process of staff engagement is structured and the vision for the service post-change is clear in your own head. If you're not sure, it is difficult to sell the concept to others. In effectively communicating your vision, you can gain trust and enthusiasm amongst others who are prepared to not only go along with the plans, and hence become *followers*, but will also be willing to engage in the implementation of change and positively influence the outcome. A lack of a clear vision (or a poorly articulated one) can lead to alienation or distrust, which can mean that changes are delayed or resisted.

**CASE STUDY**

Jane wanted to change the way patients were managed in the imaging department so that rather than all primary-care referrals being given an appointment for their X-ray, she wanted to introduce an open-access service where patients could attend when it was convenient. She had seen how this worked elsewhere, but even as a senior clinician, she did not have the authority to make such a change locally. Instead, she called all the team leaders, other clinical leads and the unit manager to a workshop to discuss her ideas. Here she shared waiting-time information, produced pathways from other facilities across the country and introduced detail of some of the strategic drivers around potential income/loss and the risks of no-change. Rather than just demanding change, she left them alone with the information to work through the pros, cons and potential actions and returned in 2 hours to an energised team who felt enabled and engaged rather than defensive. Firm plans were established, and each member of the group took away personal actions. The open access service was implemented within 2 months of the workshop to both clinical and patient appreciation.

## REFLECTION

- What was Jane's vision?

- What did Jane do to share her vision and influence others (without imposing future direction on them)?

- What information (and/or evidence) helped to support the vision?

- Who outside of the imaging department would she need to influence?

- What next steps aided the positive outcome?

- In your own department, what change would you like to see? What steps could you put in place to move towards achieving that vision?

# Understanding Cultural Diversity

Healthcare improvement, whether large or small scale, is often focussed on changes to process or role to improve the efficiency and/or delivery of current practices. These changes are sometimes described as cultural, with *culture* being defined as either a 'metaphor' for the social being of an organisation or an 'attribute' capable of manipulation and transformation (Scott et al. 2003). Whichever definition is used, the personal and professional beliefs of individuals are influenced by the culture and cultural diversity of an organisation or network. Traditional views of diversity relate to ethnicity or religion, and in the context of health care both have influence over the types of intervention offered or received, for example the use of blood products or pregnancy choices. However, other cultures (and subcultures) are at play in the health- and social-care arena, including occupation and speciality. Your team may include different occupational groups or professions such as doctor, nurse, allied health profession (therapist), support worker or manager. Each of these has historic hierarchical and gender imbalances which are increasingly being challenged and eroded, but need to be recognised. Rogers (2012) suggests that styles vary between professions, with doctors resisting collaboration as they are trained to function independently and are not afraid of making decisions autonomously. In contrast, nurses prefer to lead by example. Even within the same occupational groups, differing responsibilities and specialties (e.g., paediatrics, surgery, primary care) can result in practitioners having varied, but equally valid, views.

It is important to identify and recognise diversity within both teams and patient groups, as these may influence openness and willingness to undertake change.

## ACTIVITY

Think about your team:

- What cultural diversity do you have (staff and/or patients)?
- How might diversity positively influence planned change?

| | |
|---|---|
| Ethnicities | |
| Religions | |
| Occupations | |
| Specialties | |

## REFLECTION

If you were extending the opening hours of an out-patient service to include weekend and/or evening sessions, what cultural issues may arise as a consequence of your staff/patient demographics?

# Identifying Skills

Whereas cultural diversity may be difficult to change, the skill diversity of a team can be readily influenced. Whether this is through training, recruitment or empowerment, the skills (and potential) of team members need to be appreciated, as this may make or break a project. To implement changes in practice requires the buy-in of a few key individuals who may engage and influence others. However, those who jump on board first are not necessarily the most influential. Understanding the composition of a team is important as knowledge of individual skills and traits can allow you to tailor information and delegate activities appropriately and with confidence. (It may be useful to revisit Chapter 4, 'Models of Communication Excellence', at this point along with Chapter 6, 'Effective Leadership of Teams'.) In relation to the proposed changes, what are going to be the key qualities desired of the people around you—good communication skills with patients or other staff, organisation skills, vision or imagination? All of these are important attributes which will be critical to success in different scenarios, but may not be relevant to all projects.

Riggo, Chaleff and Lipman-Blumen (2008, pp. 7–11) describe how, as individuals become followers of a leader, they adopt different styles including the passive *Sheep*, the positive *Yes-people*, the negative *Alienated*, the political *Pragmatist* and the thinking *Star follower*. Further, they suggest that teams made up of all *Yes-people* tend to be loyal and dependable but are unlikely to include independent critical thinkers who truly engage. In relation to your team, there will be a range of skills and working styles which may be complementary and necessary for effective service delivery.

## REFLECTION

1. In your team/project—what 'individual types' do you recognise?

2. Are there any gaps? Where might you go to recruit into these gaps?

# Culture and Values

So you now know yourself (Chapter 2), your team (Chapter 6), and their attributes, but how about the organisation? Leadership styles will need to vary depending on the organisation's culture. Often no matter how hard an individual tries, if the proposed change is in opposition to the values of the employer(s), then it will not succeed. This is even more important where changes in practice are required to influence across organisational boundaries.

So how do you understand your organisation's values and culture? In health care, the values tend to be somewhat similar and shared with the patient at the centre of planning and decision making. However, certain sectors will vary, particularly in private practice, where financial influence will have a bearing on decision making. One of the most well-known and researched theories on organisations is the Competing Values Framework (CVF) initially proposed by Quinn and Rohrbaugh (1983) and refined by Quinn (1988) and others to define organisational values and culture. In their framework, an organisation's focus may be toward internal or external markets, whilst the preference for change is seen as flexible or stable. Many have used this framework and subsequent analysis materials to evaluate workplaces and such evaluation can be useful to understand culture, whether at the department or organisational level. For examples, see Ovseiko and Buchan (2012); Lin et al. (2012); and Mohr, Young and Burgess (2012). If you are experiencing challenge within your workplace in terms of historical or entrenched beliefs or processes, then an analysis of the CVF, even at a superficial level, may provide an insight into the approaches required to engage and influence change.

## REFLECTION

1. What is your department's practice?

   a. *Outward looking*: focussing on customers (patients) or commissioners

   b. *Inward looking*: focussed on staff

c. *Flexible*: regularly reviewing and changing processes

d. *Stable*: focussed on control and standards

2. How does this provide insight into how best to present your vision and influence those around you?

# Individual Leadership Values

More recently, the CVF has been developed to assist individuals in identifying their leadership behaviour and may also be a useful tool to examine roles within a change environment. Many authors (Belasen and Frank 2008; Lawrence, Lenk and Quinn 2009 and others) have sought to identify traits and behaviours using diagramatic representation of the CVF, for example, see Figure 11.1.

There are many personality profile programmes available based upon CVF and similar approaches, a number of which are free online. We would recommend that you explore how you approach a problem and identify what your values are (see Chapter 2) and what roles from Figure 11.1 you may have to fulfil to drive any changes you have identified. A thorough exploration of the issues prior to action will ensure a well-prepared, well-considered change process more likely to lead to a successful outcome.

Consensus is that those individuals who lie between the flexibility and internal axes (see Figure 11.1) are focussed on collaboration

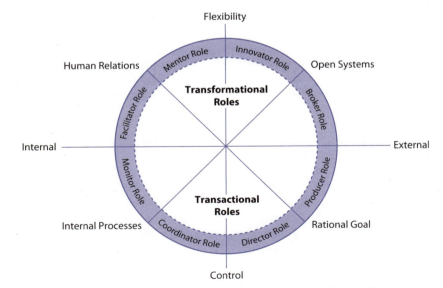

**FIGURE 11.1** Competing values framework at an individual level (Belasen and Frank 2008).

(human relations) and motivating a workforce, whereas those aligning with a creative (open systems) approach rely on communication to bring about change. Both these quadrants describe transformational roles focussed on change. Other leadership styles are more appropriately termed transactional and are focussed on control (internal processes) and individuals with these traits will often find themselves in a project manager or systems maintenance role. The final quadrant (rational goal) encompasses competitive skills with individuals who drive change and are goal focussed.

## Summary

Bringing about changes in practice can be immensely rewarding, but it is not without challenges. The effective leader can examine opportunities for innovation and improvement and enact change, bringing with them an empowered and energetic team.

Working across professional and organisational boundaries provides a chance to interact with new people and teams, but sensitivity to, and respect for, their cultures and values are required to gain cooperation. It is this genuine desire to connect with, and understand, all perspectives which generates great leadership.

## References

Belasen, A., and N. Frank. 2008. Competing values leadership: Quadrant roles and personality traits. *Leadership and Organisation Development Journal* 29: 127–43.

Denning, S. 2007. *The secret language of leadership: How leaders inspire through narrative.* San Francisco: Wiley.

Kings Fund. 2012. *Leadership and engagement for improvement in the NHS: Together we can.* Report from the Kings Fund Leadership Review. London: The Kings Fund.

Knippenberg, D. V., and M. A. Hogg, eds. 2004. *Leadership and power: Identity processes in groups and organizations.* London: Sage.

Lawrence, K. A., P. Lenk, and R. E. Quinn. 2009. Behavioural complexity in leadership: The psychometric properties of a new instrument to measure behavioural repertoire. *The Leadership Quarterly* 20: 87–102.

Lin, B. Y.-J., T. T. H. Wan, C.-P. C. Hsu, F. R. Hung, C. W. Wan, and C. C. Lin. 2012. Relationships of hospital-based emergency department culture to work satisfaction and intent to leave of emergency physicians and nurses. *Health Service Management Research* 25: 68–77.

Mohr, D. C., G. J. Young, and J. F. Burgess. 2012. Employee turnover and operational performance: The moderating effect of group-oriented organisational culture. *Human Resource Management Journal* 22: 216–33.

Northouse, P. G. 2007. *Leadership: Theory and practise.* 4th ed. Thousand Oaks, CA: Sage.

Ovseiko, P. V., and A. M. Buchan. 2012. Organizational culture in an academic health center: An exploratory study using a competing values framework. *Academic Medicine* 87: 709–18.

Quinn, R. E. 1988. *Beyond rational management: Mastering the paradoxes and competing demands of high performance*. San Francisco: Jossey-Bass.

Quinn, R. E., and J. A. Rohrbaugh. 1983. A spatial model of effectiveness criteria: Towards a competing values approach to organizational analysis. *Management Science* 29: 363–77.

Riggo, R. E., I. Chaleff, and J. Lipman-Blumen. 2008. *The art of followership*. San Francisco: Jossey-Bass.

Rogers, R. 2012. Leadership communication styles: A descriptive analysis of health care professionals. *Journal of Healthcare Leadership* 4: 47–57.

Scott. T., R. Mannion, H. T. O. Davies, and M. N. Marshall. 2003. Implementing culture change in healthcare: Theory and practise. *International Journal for Quality in Health Care* 15: 111–18.

# 12 Learning from Experience

Denise Bancroft

Moving away from leading change, this chapter explores how leaders can continually grow and develop in their own learning journey to continually strive for excellence in leadership.

Most learners would recognise that they learn from experience, but how does that learning happen and how can it be utilised? What thought processes lead to the absorption of new information, the transformation into new concepts and mental models and ultimately new ways of behaviour?

Conclusions based on both experience and research indicate that many learners approach 'on-the-job' or experiential learning on a superficial level and so gain little benefit from it. This may be due to a lack of skills in interpreting the experience and extracting the learning from it, or just because they fail to reflect on the experience due to a lack of time. In a study conducted in the UK with new managers (Bancroft 2000), they stated unanimously that sharing experience from on-the-job learning was, for them, the most beneficial way of learning. So it seems evident that gaining skills in turning experience into new concepts and practical behaviours, which can be shared, would increase the learning potential of every new manager or leader.

David Kolb (1984) is probably the most influential writer on experiential learning, and he created a model which clearly differentiates the stages of learning, where the learner:

1. Has an experience, whether that is actively engaging in an activity or by reading or observing new information

2. Then reflects on what happened during the experience and comes up with some conclusions

3. Filters those conclusions through their own experience, beliefs and values and develops new concepts regarding that experience

4. Applies those new concepts to a different situation

Kolb calls these stages Concrete Experience, Reflective Observation, Abstract Conceptualisation, and Active Experimentation.

However, in reality, many learners only engage in reflection and abstract conceptualisation in a very superficial way. For example, they may have an interaction with a staff member that went badly, reflect that it was a disaster and conclude that they have terrible leadership skills, which will influence any future similar interactions they have with staff. Or, if it went well, they may decide to use exactly the same approach as a positive model in a future interaction and yet have a complete disaster. This may be because the situation has changed, and their approach, although previously successful, hasn't adapted to the parameters of the new situation. The importance of context is well established in leadership literature (Kempster 2006).

Many learning models have been based on Kolb's work, and a cycle of reflective learning can be developed using Kolb's cycle as a base.

Kolb's concrete experience stage can be replaced with experiencing or encountering new learning, thus broadening the range of learning 'input' opportunities to apply to any type of learning. The crucial element in the whole cycle is intentionally reflecting on the learning and, from this, creating new mental constructs.

## Reflective Learning

A number of writers have investigated the area of reflective learning. Donald Schön (1983) suggested that the individual learns by both reflection-in-action and reflection-on-action. The first of the two is when learners reflect on their actions during the experience, and the second is when learners reflect on their actions afterwards. Reflection-in-action occurs when learners encounter a new situation and discover that their 'tacit' knowledge, or how they have learned to 'do things', does not give them any direction because they have not encountered this situation before, so they are forced to develop a strategy while dealing with the situation. Reflection-on-action is when learners consciously reflect on their actions after the incident.

Argyris and Schön's (1974) single- and double-loop learning theory is based on the premise that single-loop learning deals with very simple basic adjustments to behaviour, whereas double-loop learning involves changes to the individual's underlying values and assumptions. So in any new situation that arises, the individual learners gain immense value from understanding their own view of the world and how it impacts on their problem-solving strategies. To illustrate the difference between the two, in a problem-solving scenario, a problem may be identified and a solution put in place that fixes that immediate problem. This is single-loop learning, where the individual learners find the best solution that fits with their governing values and processes. In double-loop learning, the wider context of the problem will be investigated, and the solution may involve changing processes or procedures at a team, departmental or organisational level. That is, many variables that surround the problem may need to be modified to prevent the situation that caused it from reoccurring. This is similar to systems thinking, which is a holistic approach to problem solving and which stresses the relationships between the systems or components of a problem that interact and relate to each other, rather than focussing on the individual components of the systems themselves. Both have value in problem solving. With double-loop learning, the context will be considered, and in systems thinking, the relationships between all the elements that make up the problem will be analysed. An effective leader will use the most appropriate strategy in practice to get the desired outcome.

So how does the learner use reflection to successfully create new mental models?

As previously discussed, the reflective and conceptualisation stages tend to be the weaker areas, so the learner needs to consciously work through the whole cycle using the following questions as a guideline.

During the reflective stage

- What did I do well?
- Why did it go well? What behaviours did I use?
- What didn't go well?
- Why didn't it go well? Which of my behaviours contributed to this?

During the abstract conceptualisation stage

- What have I learned from what went well?
- How can I use this knowledge to build a new mental model for similar situations?
- What have I learned from what didn't go well?
- What can I do differently?
- How does that fit with how I do things?
- Are there some general principles that I can adapt to different situations?

## REFLECTION

Think back to an event which you would have liked to have handled even more successfully. Work through the previous list of questions to create a new mental model to use in future similar situations. Then repeat the activity with a situation or event that you did handle successfully, and revise the new strategy so that it can be adapted to a variety of other situations.

## Summary

It is surmised from the wealth of research conducted in this area that learning during an experience is instantaneous and context specific. It also suggests that although individuals state that learning occurs during any new experience, the most beneficial aspect of 'learning from experience' appears to be the process of reflecting on real experience and turning this intuitive, insightful learning into understanding, thereby enabling the learner to adapt a previously successful solution and apply it to other situations. And for some people, this can be even further enhanced through conversation with others, which will be discussed in the next section.

# Learning from Critical Incidents

Now that individual learners have reflected on the value of reflective learning, they might ask themselves, 'What new experiences would be the most valuable to reflect on?' The answer is the experiences that have the most significance to them. These may be termed *critical incidents*, or to lessen confusion about those only referring to negative events, they are often referred to as *significant learning events*, and again there has been much research conducted in the area. The foremost writer is John Flanagan (1954), who originally developed the critical incident technique. Flanagan defines this as

> a set of procedures for collecting direct observations of human behaviour in such a way as to facilitate their potential usefulness in solving practical problems and developing broad psychological principles. (From Easterby-Smith et al. 1991, p. 83)

The technique described by Flanagan involves having subjects write answers to written questions relating to critical incidents in order to gain descriptions of effective and ineffective behaviours. Flanagan's technique involves (a) subjects who had experienced the behaviour or (b) subjects who had observed the behaviour in others and were familiar with the critical incident. These observers are then asked to report on specific observable influences which have led to a positive or negative influence on that behaviour. The contextual element of the behaviour is then described along with the consequences of the behaviour, and these are used to explain what led the observer to decide that the behaviour was positive or negative.

In the context of this chapter, a critical incident is defined as an unfamiliar situation (a situation that the learner has no personal experience of dealing with in the past) that requires a successful solution and is critical to the learner's performance in the role.

In analysing a critical incident, the learner should consider:

- Where and when the incident occurred (who was involved, what else was happening?)

- The contextual elements which led to the behaviour of those involved (their values, attitudes, knowledge, and skills)

- The outcome and consequences of the incident

### REFLECTION

- Identify a past critical incident in your own practice and use the preceding prompts to analyse it.

- How did this process help you to explore that event?

- What new learning have you gained as a result?

- How can you incorporate this learning into your own CPD (continuing professional development) record?

## Using Critical Incidents to Analyse Team Performance

Flanagan's process can be illustrated by exploring multiple critical incidents such as a leader might do to examine team performance. Flanagan later suggests a 10-step approach (1957) in Easterby-Smith et al. (1991, p. 83) for analysing critical incidents, which focuses on gaining objective information. This approach would be useful in analysing critical incidents experienced by a team over a set period of time.

I created a nine-step approach adapted from Flanagan's model, which I used in analysing qualitative information.

1. Select a frame of reference and decide on broad general categories.

2. Create tentative headings or questions you want to discuss.

3. Group similar statements together under headings.

4. Create new headings for statements that haven't been classified under any existing group.

5. When all statements have been classified, create tentative definitions for each group or classification.

6. Decide the levels of specificity that have been generated and that you will use.

7. Redefine them if necessary.

8. Table each classification and definition.

9. Arrange for a check to be made on the classifications by an independent party.

The case study below demonstrates how this process could be used in practice; although the group studied was not a team, they were in similar roles.

## Using Critical Incident Analysis

In 1997 I was tasked with developing a new strategy for developing leaders, so I decided to research how new leaders learned from on-the-job experience. I developed in-depth, semi-structured interviews using a questioning technique based on Flanagan's (1957, in Easterby-Smith et al. 1991) critical incident technique. New leaders were asked to identify and describe two significant incidents that had occurred in their current role which were critical to their success and which they personally dealt with.

The sample group of 22, had, within the previous 2 years, been promoted into their first leadership role.

I chose this technique because, by guiding the subjects through a series of in-depth questions, they were able to reflect systematically on their experience and develop some conclusions as to why things had developed the way they had. But more importantly, they were able to see the relationship between their behaviour and the outcome of the situation. This enabled them to develop some new concepts and strategies.

I have included an example of my analysis of the following categories to illustrate Blackhurst's (1997) summary of Flanagan's steps (1957, in Easterby-Smith et al. 1991). For brevity, I have only selected one of my broad categories and defined it down to step 6:

Step 1.  Broad categories, e.g., reflection strategies

Step 2.  Critical incidents, e.g., all descriptions that described how subjects reflected were sorted under this category

Step 3.  Tentative categories, e.g., manager initiated, self-initiated

Step 4.  Further categories, e.g., directed reflection, coached reflection

Step 5.  Self-explanatory

Step 6.  Definitions of Levels 1–6 reflection strategies

The next section will focus on reflective approaches individuals could take to increase the learning they can extract from their own experiences.

# Using Critical Incidents to Analyse Individual Behaviour

In analysing one's own behaviour, the individual may reflect on a personal critical incident:

- To identify the underlying behaviours that lead to its outcome
- To improve their practice
- To solve a problem by identifying how it could be improved or avoided

The basis of this process is 'reflection on action' (Schön 1983), or thinking about how they handled the situation, what they did, which of their behaviours were constructive and which were not, and then developing a framework to strengthen positive behaviours and eliminate negative ones. To do this, once a learner has chosen a critical incident to reflect on, the next step is to work through the list of questions already discussed under reflective learning to identify and strengthen positive behaviours.

In deciding to use critical incident analysis, the learner should not forget to also examine successful incidents. A lot of valuable learning can be extracted from a positive example, yet these are often ignored, and so learners become flummoxed when a solution that worked well before is less effective the next time they use it. The key is not only to extract the constructive behaviours, but also to reflect on how to transfer those good principles to another situation.

# Peer Mentoring and Social Learning

Up till this point in the chapter, the emphasis has been on individuals learning from their own experience; however, the value of sharing experience and learning with others cannot be understated.

This is where the experienced mentor, leader, or peer group can have a major impact in guiding the reflection process and enabling the learner to develop the skills necessary to gain new insights from their own experience.

There are many benefits to shared learning:

- The joy of sharing experience
- Networking opportunities

- Support from others
- Recognition that colleagues in similar roles face similar challenges, which tends to increase confidence in their own ability

The principle upon which peer learning is built is that in helping each other to solve problems, people learn to help themselves. According to Revans (1982), this group learning helps the individual by providing support, constructive criticism and advice. The source of the learning is personal experience and re-interpretation of that experience as opposed to the more traditional input of new information by 'experts'. The dynamics of this group learning is that interaction with other learners creates new insights into problems and generates ideas. It allows each member to benefit from and acknowledge group and individual expertise, not only from receiving input from the whole team, but also from framing their own experience to share with others.

Because this type of learning is live 'learning by doing', learners have to be committed to it and cannot simply pay lip service as is possible in other types of learning.

This group learning, initially termed a *learning set*, now often termed *action learning sets*, observed the following format:

- Participants choose a real problem to work on that is relevant to their work role.
- Regular meetings are arranged for a finite period of time.
- The group or 'set' reviews each individual's progress regularly.

From this type of learning, peer group mentoring has now evolved, which has many of the same principles, but the individuals do not have a single set problem. They choose to work on an issue or situation they are currently facing.

- It enables them to work in a way that encapsulates many of the identified strategies that help adults to learn.
- It allows them to use their own experience, using relevant 'live' scenarios that have a practical application.
- It allows them to work at their own pace.
- It gives them time to discuss with others but also reflect individually.
- It allows them to design their own learning and interact with peers.

This group learning is not bound by regulations or syllabus or any teacher-led instruction. It is this freedom that allows the learners to approach their learning in creative and diverse ways that are appropriate to the situation and the group itself. It also means that whilst strictly observing the confidentially of group makeup, members may come from any discipline, which in turn adds new perspectives and brings diversity.

However, peer group learning should be approached in a structured and organised way. Group members must be committed to the peer group, because there will be times when they do not feel comfortable to be challenged, yet they still have a role to play in giving constructive feedback to other members of the group. To be successful and achieve their potential as a learning medium, peer groups should have a static membership who meet regularly and follow the same structure each time they meet. Each participant must have a very clear idea of what their role is and the self-discipline to carry it out.

Typical structure of a peer group meeting:

- A facilitator and a timekeeper are chosen at the start of each session.
- Each member of the group gives a cathartic overview and states if they have an issue they want to share.
- The group then chooses the issue or issues they want to work on for that session.
- The owner of each issue advises the group how long they will spend on each issue.
- The owner of the issue tells the group what type of feedback they should give. This could be:

Group gives examples of similar experiences.

Group sensitively challenges assumptions.

Group gives positive feedback.

Group role-plays situation.

Group questions owner for greater clarification.

- The group then offers feedback rather than advice, following whichever feedback style the owner has requested.
- Owner does not comment but listens and chooses what is most useful.
- The owner of the issue thanks the group.
- At the end of the session, the group shares how they are now feeling.

Peer group mentoring, once seen mainly in the education world as a part of the student curriculum, is now gaining wide acceptance in the business world and across health care, both within organisations, across organisations, and amongst professional groups.

## REFLECTION

Consider your own colleagues and peers and who you could invite to join a peer mentoring group.

It may be helpful to read one of the many books on mentoring, such as David Clutterbuck's (1991) *Everyone Needs a Mentor*, to help in setting up a peer mentoring group. There are also many online groups and resources.

## Summary

This chapter has provided some insights into how healthcare professionals can learn from work-based experiences, and has provided some practical tools to use both individually and in groups. I encourage you to engage in reflective learning at a whole new level, exploring options both individually and with peers, to enhance not only your own effectiveness, but also the quality of service delivery possible.

## References

Argyris, C., and D. A. Schön. 1974. *Theory in practise: Increasing professional effectiveness*. San Francisco: Jossey-Bass.

Bancroft, D. 2000. An investigation into managerial on-the-job learning. Master's thesis. Henley, UK.

Blackhurst, A. 1997. *TAM/UKAT National Technology Competency Identification study*. University of Kentucky Assistive Project.

Clutterbuck, D. 1991. *Everyone needs a mentor*. New York: Hyperion Books.

Easterby-Smith, M., R. Thorpe, and A. Lowe. 1991. *Management research: An introduction*. London: Sage.

Flanagan, J. C. 1954. (described in *Psychological Bulletin*), 51 (4), July.

Kempster, S. 2006. Leadership learning through lived experience: A process of apprenticeship? *Journal of Management & Organization* 12 (1): 4–22.

Kolb, D. A. 1984. *Experiential learning: Experience as the source of learning and development*. Englewood Cliffs, NJ: Prentice Hall.

Revans, R. W. 1982. *The origins and growth of action learning*. Kent, UK: Chartwell-Bratt Ltd.

Schön, D. A. 1983. *The reflective practitioner: How professionals think in action*. New York: Basic Books.

## Additional Reading

Argyris, C. 1995. Action science and organisational learning. *Journal of Managerial Psychology* 10 (6): 20–26.

Bandura, A. 1977. *Social learning theory*. Englewood Cliffs, NJ: Prentice Hall.

Boud, D., R. Cohen, and D. Walker, eds. 1993. *Using experience for learning.* Buckingham, England: The Society for Research into Higher Education & Open University Press.

Boyatzis, R. E., and D. A. Kolb. 1995. From learning styles to learning skills: The executive skills profile. *Journal of Managerial Psychology* 10 (5): 3–15.

Brookfield, S. 1990. Using critical incidents to explore learner's assumptions. In *Fostering critical reflection in adulthood*, ed. J. Meizirow & Assoc. San Francisco: Jossey-Bass.

Hergenhahn, B. R. 1982. *An introduction to the theories of learning.* 2nd ed. Englewood Cliffs, NJ: Prentice Hall.

Knowles, M. 1984. *The adult learner: A neglected species.* Houston, TX: Gulf.

Marsick, V. J. 1990. Action learning and reflection in the workplace. In *Fostering critical reflection in adulthood*, ed. J. Meizirow & Assoc., 23–46. San Francisco: Jossey-Bass.

Schön, D. A. 1990. *Educating the reflective practitioner.* 1st ed. San Francisco: Jossey-Bass.

# 13 Coaching and Empowering Others

Joseph Quinn, Anna McNaughton and Suzanne Henwood

The previous chapters have explored various components of leadership and demonstrated the enormity of the task when the role is taken seriously to effect positive change and future possibility. We know that working in the healthcare industry can be incredibly rewarding. However, at the same time, it is also both emotionally and physically demanding, so ensuring that practitioners have healthy proactive support and development opportunities is vital. The challenges in the healthcare environment have increased over the years, with a more rapid rate of change, increasing regulation, the need for compliance with targets and directives, and rising expectations from patients alongside greater public scrutiny.

Before we explore support in more depth, it is important to clarify the difference between professional development and support versus the need for therapeutic intervention. Many organisations support and encourage staff to access counselling or employee assistance programmes for personal or work-related issues that require short-term intervention or counselling which may be of a more therapeutic nature. This tends to be more of a reactive response to situations in one's work/life. Conversely, practitioners also require more professional and personal development in practice, including mentoring, professional supervision and coaching, which is what we will be outlining in this chapter. These can be both proactive and reactive and often allow healthcare professionals to maintain and increase their clinical and leadership skills: They are activities undertaken by strong effective leaders who want to make even more of an impact.

## REFLECTION

- What are your experiences of these development opportunities (mentoring, supervision and coaching) from either a receiving or providing perspective?

- What has worked well for you (and how did it help), and what may be useful to explore afresh?

# Mentoring, Supervision and Coaching: Understanding the Difference

Mentoring and supervision are quite common in health care, so this chapter focusses specifically on coaching in more detail to provide some new practical perspectives and possible applications for your clinical practice and leadership roles in a healthcare context.

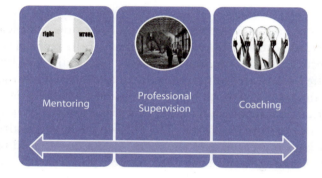

## Supervision

Supervision is often a reflective process where someone has an experienced practitioner to support them in reflecting and working on their professional practice. Bishop (2006) suggests that the aims of supervision are to safeguard standards of practice, to develop the individual both professionally and personally, and to promote excellence in healthcare practice. In most healthcare settings, professional supervision allows someone to look at their practice and explore challenges and issues that may arise both on a case-by-case and overall perspective. Having someone with whom to discuss the details about cases, strategies and approaches is seen as a vital part of improving clinical competence and effectiveness while also enhancing the overall well-being of the health professional (Lyth 2000; Yegdich 1999). Different perspectives of supervision sometimes split it into clinical supervision and professional supervision or line management supervision. It is important to be clear about the purpose and boundaries of supervision when establishing such a relationship.

# Mentoring

Mentoring often involves a more senior or experienced practitioner who serves as a role model in support of a younger or more junior member of staff in an area or technique. The use of mentoring in health care is also often one where students on placement are supported by a mentor who they can shadow to see how theory and practice are integrated. The mentor typically supports them as they work their way up to handling a small workload in the workplace. This relationship is definitely one where the mentor is more of a discipline or technical expert, which allows mentors to share their knowledge and experience. It is worth considering that mentoring with, or shadowing a senior leader, can be a great learning opportunity for new or emerging leaders to role model or fine-tune their own leadership skills. Who might you ask to mentor you to take your skills to the next level?

# Coaching

Coaching is an altogether different process. A coach helps someone to identify and understand any issues and areas of desired change and then helps them to utilise their own beliefs, skills and resources to achieve their own success. It is very client driven, and a coach is there to help individuals reach their own potential by supportively exploring issues at depth and asking questions to probe and stretch their awareness and understanding while opening up options to pursue.

This can be achieved through a range of strategies and approaches, e.g., GROW model (Goal, Reality, Opportunity, Wrap-up), Neuro-Linguistic Programming (NLP), multiple Brain Integration Techniques (mBIT), business or executive coaching, and career coaching. It is important to research the appropriate style of coaching to suit your own preferences and needs, as well as ensuring you seek a qualified and experienced coach to maximise the return on your investment.

## What Is Coaching and How Can I Apply It to My Practice?

At one level, coaching involves a set of specific skills and techniques to foster personal and professional development on the part of the *coachee*, but it is also a process of 'awakening and enabling'. The growth gained through coaching continues to evolve over many weeks, months and years because of the level of ownership secured by the coachee right from the outset. The coach, not being a mentor (a person with greater competence in the same area who shares more expert advice), (a) assists coachees in identifying where they are now (pacing current experience), (b) works with them to identify where they want to be (leading towards desired future), and (c) assists them in exploring how they can make the necessary changes to get to that new desired point.

Coaching has a strong outcome focus: Every action will be guided toward the overall objective and the use of questions, more than answers, which plays a significant part in allowing the person being coached to move forward with a purpose while remaining in overall control of the direction of travel.

Just take a moment to reflect on this: How different is your own thinking when you are simply given an answer from the perspective of another person versus being *asked* a question which challenges you to consider your own perspective?

Coaching is not about giving the answers, it is about helping coachees to identify the right questions and then supporting them in finding their own answers. Empowering language is a particularly powerful coaching tool, so coaches take care with language to ensure that they are congruent in their interactions with clients, ready to back up any conversation with action and modelling. Conversational change can happen with simple changes in the coach's language, such as swapping 'but' for 'and' or 'yet', which can quickly reframe a previously difficult situation. For example, 'I have not managed to resolve that situation (yet)'. By adding 'yet' to that sentence, it opens up the possibility that the situation will be resolved in the future, which will change the mind-set and enable new options to be considered. Coaching is also about people identifying their goals and working through obstacles, to be future focussed in a positive way, fully accessing the resources available to them both internally and externally to optimise their success.

## Obstacles

Whilst being outcome focussed is important, the journey to achieve those outcomes is of paramount importance. Life is not always as simple as agreeing to complete a goal and suddenly finding that it has been achieved (the adage 'Be careful what you wish for' comes to mind). As humans, we are thankfully, and also regrettably, much more complex than we think and often encounter unexpected obstacles to the goals we set, requiring us to be flexible in our approach to goal attainment.

It's worth bearing in mind that just because a goal was not achieved according to our original plan, this may not mean that we did not achieve it. Look at the learning we may have gained, which may have led us to a whole new direction of gaining a great deal more than we first thought. Coaching then can enable practitioners to identify positive learning from experience, which may otherwise have been overlooked, making it an even more valuable process to invest in.

So what can prevent us from achieving a goal we set our hearts and minds on? For some, that is the silver question with the golden answer. There are two main sets of obstacles:

*Exterior*. These are things which we see as totally outside of our control, such as a change in the system, budget or other resource constraints, personality differences, a decision from above, health policy, agency targets, etc.

*Interior*: Our own thoughts and feelings toward the goal/actions, such
as our self-belief and the belief in others, how much we value the
goal and are therefore motivated by it, our personality, how we
view the significance of the goal in context, etc. Another interior
obstacle sometimes seen is *secondary gain*. This is simply the case
where continuing to have a barrier/problem is more beneficial to
the person than to remove it. For example, a disorganised person may
not want to become organised because that would mean having to do
more work. Or someone may sabotage promotion prospects by holding
an unresourceful or unhelpful belief in their own abilities because they
want to have fewer responsibilities or work fewer hours.

Coaches require practical and effective language tools to tease out the 'reality'
of the goal (and any obstacles) and to explore what would enable success as
well as what may derail the entire process, which is what we will focus on in
a moment. As well as having the language skills, it would be useful to have a
logical system to use in moving through each area of goal setting.

## REFLECTION

Think of a current goal you would like to achieve. Take a moment to consider
your top four internal barriers and the top four external barriers—write them in a
list. Are they 'real' or 'perceived' barriers?

Now review each one in light of how 'real' they actually are. You may have
barriers which are simply based on your perception of what you believe to be
true as opposed to the objective reality of what actually is true. For example,
I may have a barrier to working with Jane because the last time I gave her
feedback, she got very defensive and told me I was totally wrong. So, from that
experience, I believe she is not someone I can work with on a project where
open communication is important.

Whilst this may have some 'reality' to it, i.e., the facts of what was said, there
remains a barrier in my mind of us working together in the future. Does the past
always equal the future? Was Jane becoming defensive because what I said
was true? Was she even being defensive, or was I being overly sensitive? Was
Jane just having a bad day? How might she have responded to someone else?.

It is vital to explore each barrier and look at it from a different perspective and
question its validity (consider using the perceptual positions tool from Chapter
3 to see the other person's perspective). Ask yourself, 'For what purpose am I still
identifying this as a barrier AND what can I now do about it to remove it?'

# 4MAT and Congruence

What experience has shown is that people who achieve their goals with
greater consistency are *aligned* to what's happening on the inside as well as
the outside. Their thoughts and feelings about the goal will be resourceful

so they can be flexible and strong in achieving it. This is what we mean as *congruent*, where our values, beliefs, attitude, decisions, etc. (neurological levels of change, see Chapter 2), are aligned and our inside processes match what we do on the outside. With any respected leader (family member or world visionary), we 'trust' that they value and believe what they are doing. If they were not as aligned on the inside with what they were doing, would they be as respected or trusted as they are now?

How differently would we have thought about the late Steve Jobs if we found out that he did not believe in his work and didn't really care about pioneering new technology? Maybe we would never even have heard about him if he did not believe in or did not value his work, as he never would have achieved a great deal without the inside strength and tenacity, flexibility, clear vision and direction.

In working with others around achieving outcomes, it is equally important that we assist them in being congruent so they know what drives the goal, what the goal is and how they believe they can make it happen. We also want to avoid goals being derailed before the outcome is reached, and therefore we explore some contingencies should any 'outside or internal' barriers arise.

The model we are about to share is called the 4MAT system and was created by Bernice McCarthy (2005) as a way to measure success in learning. The 4MAT is based on four simple questions which are used to gain greater congruence after first identifying the goal:

*Why*: For what purpose do I want to achieve this goal; what will happen as a result of this being achieved? This identifies the motivation of 'why' the person is doing this in the first place. In some cases, the goal may have been assigned or it is predominantly for someone else. It is then important for the individual to also find a 'personal' reason/benefit for achieving this goal: 'What's In It For Me (WIIFM)'.

*What*: This is where we explore the contents of the goal: What actually is the goal itself and the breakdown of each part required to make it happen? What would the success of the goal look and feel like?

*How*: With the 'why' and 'what' answered, we now have gained the awareness and clarity we need to make it happen, and so we create a plan of action here: the gates we need to walk through to take us to our goal, starting with a clear first step.

*What if*: This is vital, as it creates the 'reality' of unexpected events (without going too extreme, of course) and prepares people to get back on track should something happen to lead them off course. Of course, unexpected events and challenges can be positive too, as it keeps us open for new opportunities along the way. It all comes down to 'how' we choose to see them.

Before you move on, take a few moments now to have a play with this yourself. Decide upon a goal and use these four questions and see how much more awareness you gain in the process. Note: You may want to use this again after you have read the next chapter on goal setting.

# Questions Are the Answer

As coaches, we explore how a few simple questions can direct clients to uncover an insight, and with a tiny tweak in their mind, they can create the most significant difference in their lives. For example, I was recently working with a senior manager in the health service who was having a list of troubles with a person in her team. She was finding it hard to motivate this individual; she was continually chasing the underperformer to submit work in on time; she found herself having to justify actions based on this person's 'hints' of poor leadership, etc.

This 'battle' needed to stop, as it was having a detrimental effect on the wider team and their performance. We could have spent a whole session exploring the detail of each part of the battle and what she had done, what she wanted to do, what would happen next, etc. However, going back to the 4MAT model, we began with a more holistic approach and talked about what was driving all of this in the first place: What was the *motivation* for the underperformer's behaviour? And so the simple question asked was, 'What is important to this person about being in the team?' My client was at a loss and could not answer. She did not know what motivated this person to be there, and yet it was obvious that the values and motivation levels were not being met, otherwise things would be very different. The manager that day went back and spoke *with* the person involved and asked that very question. What came from this discussion was that the person found it very difficult to work in a new open-plan office and worked a great deal better on an independent basis. So a compromise was reached where this person was initially given part of a project to do independently, then reporting back to the wider team to discuss and implement. The change was significant for all those involved, allowing the team to move beyond what had been perceived as a negative stuck state.

## Congruent Questions

One of the first components of any coaching session is to specify the desired outcome. However, the process of actually verbalising and identifying what you actually want can be surprisingly difficult, and a key role of a coach is to help you define your goal(s):

'What specifically do you want?' (Delve down into greater specificity if needed.)

'How will you know when the outcome has been a success?'

'What will happen as a result of this?'

'What won't happen as a result of this?'

'What will happen if this doesn't happen?'

'What won't happen if this doesn't happen?'

Another important step is to identify why any change is desired. This will enable individuals to understand and enhance their motivation to action, i.e., you need to want it enough (linking values to action). This generates your purpose, your reason for achieving the goal, which will be your constant guide as you achieve it.

'What's important to you (others/us/them) about achieving this?'

'What else is important to you about achieving this?' (Chunk Laterally)*

'What's important to you about that?' (Chunk Up)

'Where does this fit within the larger context?'

'What's your overall purpose for wanting this achieved?'

Only then is it time to define the 'what'. This step involves driving clarity and conviction (exploring beliefs: both resourceful and unresourceful or unhelpful).

'What do you think about this being achieved?' 'What's your opinion?'

'What do others think?' 'What "may" be their opinion?'

'What's good about this being achieved?'

'What's not so good about this being achieved?'

'What roadblocks may spring up along the way?'

'What's your view about those roadblocks?'

Once the 'what' is clear, you can move on to the 'how': identifying actions and planning.

'What's needed now to make this work?'

---

* 'Chunking' is an NLP term which enables people to work at different levels of abstraction. 'Chunking Up' moves thinking out of fine detail into wider concepts and 'Chunking Down' moves from abstract generality to specific detail. To 'Chunk Laterally' is what we might know as lateral thinking, broadening the thoughts and applications possible, which may help to move someone out of a stuck state.

'What are the specific actions needed to make this happen?'

'How will these be measured?'

'Who will do what and by when?'

'How will you measure your progress?'

'Where's a logical place to begin?'

'What additional skills are/may be needed?'

A further step which it is important to consider is the 'what if', where we help the coachee to identify any potential barriers and solutions and how to overcome them.

'What may interfere with this goal?'

'How will you get around/through these roadblocks?'

'What happens if this goal is not completed on time?'

'What's next after this goal is achieved?'

'Who might also be affected by this change? Is it possibly detrimental to anyone else involved and how can that be handled respectfully?'

## ACTIVITY

Return to your goal and use these questions with another person and ask them to take you (and your goal) through these questions to gain even greater awareness and clarity. You can, of course, ask yourself these questions, although you may notice even more benefits in asking someone else to guide you through.

## CASE STUDY

### Making the Most of Coaching

Mary was an experienced nurse who, when under pressure, could sometimes be quite abrupt, to the point that some people thought she was rude. After several complaints, her manager had a chat with her and explored how Mary could change her behaviour. Mary realised that this was standing in the way of her having any leadership opportunities, so she was keen to address how she came across, as it was not her intention to be rude. After several coaching sessions, Mary understood what triggered her behaviours and had strategies to employ to help her avoid coming across in that way.

Coaching is something that people want to participate in, but not as part of a disciplinary or a forced activity; that's an entirely different beast. Coaching is all about you being fully engaged in the process and making the most of the sessions and reflecting on them to maximise results. Coaching, if effective, is not done to you; rather, it is something that you choose and embrace as you move from current state to desired state. To maximise the benefits of coaching, one might consider:

- Being open to coaching
- Being honest with yourself and your coach about all of the issues
- Trusting your coach, the process and yourself—you know yourself the best
- Taking action—having awareness is half the challenge; acting on it is the other half
- Being nice to yourself: showing yourself compassion
- Wanting to be even more effective/successful (or whatever outcome you want to substitute here)

## Tips for Selecting a Good Coach

- Look for a good fit—someone that you feel you can engage with and understand with a practical and down-to-earth approach.
- Don't opt for someone who is too easy; you want someone who will be challenging yet supportive, someone who will stretch you and help you achieve your goals.
- Find out about the reputation and credentials of your coach. Ensure that the candidate has some experience in the world and has a proven track record in coaching or associated people development. Ask about accreditation and membership in professional bodies, and seek recommendations from people you trust.

## Questions to Ask a Prospective Coach

- How long have you been a coach?
- What type of people and issues do you deal with?
- Describe the coaching process you follow.
- What do you expect of me as the coachee?
- What can I expect of you as the coach?
- How do you measure results/success?
- What tools/strategies do you have in your coaching toolkit?
- Logistic questions: cost, location, format (face to face, Skype, phone, etc.), length of session, qualifications, membership of professional bodies, etc.

# What If?

*What if I don't like the coach?* You don't have to see a coach if you don't like him or her. Saying that, it's important to reflect on what the issue is, e.g., 'Is it the coach or me?' Perhaps the coach struck an issue that you are avoiding, and by saying you don't like the coach, you don't have to deal with the issue. Just like with other healthcare decisions, you are entitled to a second opinion, so it's wise to meet with (or at least speak to) a coach beforehand to see if there is a good fit or not. Good coaches will be open to discussion around issues like this.

*What if I don't like what the coach is saying?* Ultimately, you have responsibility for your life and decisions—and the consequences of these. Explore the conversation and your reasons for not liking the coach's suggestions. This in itself may be a really useful discussion in a coaching environment.

*What if there is a conflict of interest?* All coaches should operate under clear guidelines, so if you think there might be an issue, it is important to discuss the practical options as soon as possible.

## Ethics and Excellence

It is important that any type of development or intervention be undertaken by practitioners with clear ethics and a code of conduct. Whether this comes from their clinical registration or professional body or from additional affiliations such as Association of Coaching, International Coaching Federation (ICF), ANLP (Association for Neuro-Linguistic Programming), etc., it is important to understand how ethics and issues are managed in a coaching or development relationship.

Dealing with issues

- Raise the issue with the practitioner or the practitioner's organisation. The coach should be open to having a discussion, as it's about your needs. There should be a clear complaint process to follow if you cannot resolve the issue directly with your coach.

- In extreme cases, it may be necessary to make a complaint to the practitioner's professional association, e.g., professional registration body, AfC (Association for Coaching), ICF (International Coaching Federation).

- If necessary, stop seeing them, but don't let this put you off finding another coach.

## Accessing Other Coaching Opportunities

In the tight current economy, many organisations struggle to have training budgets for the prerequisite and mandatory training, let alone for what some perceive as the luxury of coaching. In this instance, there are several options above and beyond self-investment:

## Peer Accountability

> Joe and his team decided that they needed to support each other with their personal development, so everyone in the team came to the team meeting with a priority for their leadership development with a specific action they wanted to undertake. All of the group shared their desired outcomes and actions planned, and they committed to call and support each other in doing this.

In a peer group, by making it real and giving permission to each other to help with accountability, people are often able to take more personal responsibility to succeed, as they know they have their own cheer squad as well as feedback team on board (refer back to Chapter 12 where peer mentoring was discussed in more detail).

## Coaching Partners

Having a coaching partner can also provide a supportive environment in workplaces and can be facilitated across departments as well as clinical practices. Having a time when you can share frustrations and suggestions with someone who understands the culture and organisation—but is distant from your actual workspace—can be a great way of providing peer support. This can be in a formal coaching session with each other, or it can be in a more supportive safe peer support model. One example of this is the use of coaching pairs within speciality groups, such as a consultant network, where peers can really understand and relate to your work context.

## Coaching Moments

Coaching moments can also be a great opportunity for leaders to develop their teams. How often during the day do we engage in interactions where we give people the answers to questions, when we could take 3–4 minutes and help them find the answer themselves? Additional training in coaching skills can be useful in developing our skills either for formal or informal training to offer this opportunity for deeper development in a practice setting.

# Summary

The value of coaching in the healthcare sector cannot be overstated, as it can add valuable skills to a leader's repertoire and also help to build the careers of emerging leaders. Awareness of how to use coaching effectively and making the most of coaching resources are vital to ensure that new and existing leaders and staff are supported in this challenging and complex industry. While it is not yet well utilised in a healthcare context, we have experienced the benefits both for ourselves and while working with healthcare leaders, and we believe it is part of the future of leadership development in health care.

# References

Bishop, V. 2006. *Clinical supervision in practise: Some questions, answers and guidelines for professionals in health and social care*. 2nd ed. London: Macmillan.

Lyth, G. 2000. Clinical supervision: A concept analysis. *Journal of Advanced Nursing* 31: 722–29.

McCarthy, B. 2005. *Teaching around the 4MAT cycle*. New York: Sage.

Yegdich, T., and A. Cushing. 1998. A historical perspective on nursing. *Australian and New Zealand Journal of Mental Health Nursing* 7: 3–24.

# 14 Setting Compelling Goals

Joe Cheal and Melody Cheal

Having now explored what leadership is and the components which contribute to leadership effectiveness, this chapter will explore putting that into action through the creation and setting of compelling goals. We will set a context and then reveal both the logical and psychological perspectives for making goals work. Added to this, we will share with you some key ideas on how to get specific, clear and motivated to maximise your success.

## Why Goals?

What would happen if we didn't have goals? Laurence Peter (1977, p. 125) suggested: 'If you don't know where you are going, you will probably end up somewhere else.' This is, of course, still true today. Without goals, we tend to drift. Of course, drifting can be a pleasant enough experience and can lead us to unexpected places. However, as a leader, a lack of goals tends to mean a lack of direction, which just happens to be one of the biggest criticisms of poor managers and leaders.[1] Without specific goals, we are unlikely to increase performance (Snyder and Lopez 2005), and we are more likely to stand still (which in a forward-moving and rapidly changing environment such as health care means that, relatively speaking, we are going backwards!).

Health professionals should be no stranger to goal setting when it comes to patient recovery and rehabilitation (e.g., Hartigan 2012; Hersh et al. 2012) and for interventions (e.g., Pearson 2012). So what do goals give us as *leaders* in the healthcare profession? Simply put, when goals are effectively set and applied, they give us direction and 'self leadership' (e.g., Neck, Nouri and Godwin 2003), motivation and a sense of purpose (e.g., Locke 1996), individual effectiveness and increased performance (e.g., Latham and Locke 2006) and a way of measuring progress. Ultimately, they help us achieve what we want to achieve, and as a leader, this means helping the organisation to be healthy and prosperous, while the patient receives excellent patient care.

# A Goal-Setting Context

## Mission–Goal–Objective

Our mission could be defined as the bigger-picture goal of the organisation (what are we really here for?). Our own goals (team and individual) will then plug into the mission. According to Chris Argyris (1994), keeping a view on our mission, as we set and action our goals, helps us to maintain 'double loop' learning (already discussed in Chapter 12). To recap: This means being aware of the purpose of our processes whilst we implement them. When we lose sight of the mission we tend to revert to 'single loop' learning, which can feel like setting goals and carrying out actions for the sake of setting goals and carrying out actions! Malott (2003) suggests that leaders who lose sight of the mission tend to micromanage, getting caught in the trap of simply carrying out actions. As healthcare professionals, it is very easy to get caught in the day-to-day service delivery to meet targets, clear lists and provide care; however, by considering 'mission' as well, a whole new layer of potential development opens up.

Our goals give us direction (what and where to) and motivation (why). Some of our goals are more important than others, and so they tend to sit in a hierarchy of priority. This hierarchy may change over time, depending on the environment, with certain goals being high priority one week and then lower priority the next. As a leader, it is helpful to be transparent and let people know that the priority of goals will likely fluctuate over time, and ensure that you keep all staff fully informed of the direction you are working towards.

Then objectives tend to be tighter, more specific, more practically based in reality and time. They need to be quantifiable, measurable and without ambiguity. Typically, objectives are functional and instructional but may not necessarily be motivational in and of themselves. In this chapter we will be suggesting a 'best of both worlds' approach by helping you to 'objectify' your goals.

## Strategic Planning and Goals

In order to be successful, a leader needs to be able to plan strategically, to look at the big picture and translate that into the real world. In simplistic terms, strategic planning requires us knowing three things: our current situation, our desired situation and an idea of how to get from one to the other. Once we have identified our current situation, we can then set goals which define where we want to be and/or how we want to be different. When we have this clear, we can determine our plan.

## REFLECTION

As a healthcare practitioner, what is it that excites you strategically—above and beyond what you do now?

Where do you want to be personally and where do you want your service/profession to be five years from now?

How would you describe where you are now and where you desire to be?

## How People Stop Themselves Achieving the Goals

Professor Richard Wiseman (2009) carried out a long-term study with over 5000 people who wanted to achieve a personal goal. By the end of the research, only 10% had achieved their goal.[2] So, before we discuss the success factors, what kinds of things do people do or not do that means they are more likely to fail? In our experience, here are a few key mistakes:

- They focus on what they *don't* want, e.g., 'We don't want to make a loss next year'.
- There is no end point or the end point is immeasurable, e.g., 'We want to raise our profile' or to 'improve quality'.
- The goal is unrealistic in some way, usually due to overly tight timescales/budgets and/or a lack of appreciation of how busy they and others are with ongoing daily workload/projects.
- There is a lack of motion/motivation or they run out of steam part way through as motivation lessens.
- The goal is too big and overwhelming, so people don't know where to start.
- There are unexpected/unforeseen barriers and unintended consequences that bring the implementation to a halt.
- There are too many other distractions and people try to 'spread themselves too thinly'.
- The contextual situation changes but no adjustment is made to the goal.

In this chapter we intend to help you prevent and/or address these issues through setting 'successful goals' that increase your likelihood of achievement.

# Successful Goals

According to Snyder and Lopez (2005), there are a number of key criteria for successful goals, including:

- *Challenge*: The goals take us beyond our 'normal' day-to-day activities, stretching us to step up and improve, developing and achieving something motivational.

- *Clarity*: The goals are understandable and understood; they give us clear direction. If you have ever been given a task to do but not been clear of what you are meant to be doing, you will know how that feels and want to make sure you help others by giving them clarity.

- *Knowledge of results*: Not only do goals need to be measurable, but there also needs to be a feedback loop within the process so people know how they are doing. If they do not know they are on track, they are, in effect, lost. So inspire others by letting them know how far they have come.

- *Value orientation*: Goals need to be tied to values, i.e., what's important. This could be on an individual and/or organisational level: Why do we have this goal? If you have ever been given a task without being told why, how motivated were you? You may have been compliant perhaps, but probably not committed. Let people know why these specific goals have been set and why they are important.

## REFLECTION

Think of a time when you were highly motivated by a goal and you achieved that goal. In relation to the criteria just discussed, how were each met in your situation?

## CASE STUDY

### A Goal for Supporting Lone Worker Nurses

In a healthcare organisation, there was a rising concern for the welfare of nurses working in the community in isolation and visiting patients in their homes. A goal was set to 'make nurses feel more supported and hence safer'. This was quantified by seeking a reduction in the amount of reported conflicts and aggressive incidents, both verbal and physical.

There was a secondary goal, which was to bring about more successful prosecutions where attacks happened, since previously, very few cases were brought to trial due to there being a lack of evidence.

continued ...

The solution put in place was to have a communication system that recorded a live audio feed of where the nurses were and what was happening. Any problems would result in the police being called immediately (when needed) from a remote base. This was done to support the nurses as well as raising the alert to their manager.

As well as a reduction in conflict, a qualitative measure was taken before and after the communication system was introduced, and nurses reported feeling safer after receiving the communication devices.

Following on from this, two unintended issues arose that had to be dealt with. The first was that in feeling safer, the nurses were sometimes taking a risk and staying in an unsafe environment. The second was that management concluded that since nurses were safer, they might no longer need a second member of staff with them, thereby also increasing the risk to the nurses.

# Goal Setting: Logical and Psychological

As the case study presented here demonstrates, when setting goals you may get what you asked for, but that might not always be what you meant. In addition, a goal may have unintended consequences. So how do we make sure we get what we really want and are prepared for unintended consequences?

Successful goal setting requires an external, objective, pragmatic perspective *and* an internal, subjective, motivational perspective. We call this the 'logical' and the 'psychological' approach to goal setting. Did the goal in the previous case study meet the 'logical' and the 'psychological' criteria? Read on.

## Logical

According to Latham and Locke (2006, 332), goals assigned by a manager 'are as effective as self-set or participatively set goals *if they are accompanied by logic or a rationale* from a manager' (our emphasis). Goals without reason or logic, whilst perhaps commanding compliance, are unlikely to engender commitment.

Traditional goal-setting approaches tend to utilise the acronym 'SMART' which has existed and persisted since at least the early 1980s (Doran 1981). Although originally designed for objective setting, SMART gives us a useful set of criteria for the externalisation of the goal (i.e., how it will manifest in the real world). Over time, the SMART acronym (e.g., specific, measurable, assignable/achievable, realistic/relevant and time related) has been adopted and adapted and written about extensively. For this reason (and due to diligence of chapter space), if you are not familiar with SMART goals and objectives, we would encourage you to explore them further.[3]

## Psychological

As well as working corporately, we also have a strong background in the field of NLP (see sidebar), where we are interested in the subjective experience of the individual. In NLP, there is an internal, 'psychological' framework for making sure goals are 'well formed' (e.g., Day and Tosey 2011), i.e., more likely to succeed. For a goal or outcome to be considered well formed, it needs to meet the following criteria, for which we (the authors) use the acronym 'POISED' (as in absolutely ready and in a state of anticipation!):

> ### NLP (Neuro-Linguistic Programming)
>
> NLP could be defined as 'the psychology of excellence and the science of change'.[4] The focus of NLP is on how what goes on in the brain (neuro) is systemically linked to the language we use (linguistic) and how we can use both language and the processes of the brain to make positive changes (programming) to our personal (subjective) experience.
>
> For more information on NLP see ANLP.org.

- *Positive*: The goal needs to be positively stated and outcome oriented to what we want rather than what we don't want. This gives us a forward-facing focus.

- *Owned*: The goal needs an owner. For individuals to take ownership of the goal (or for their part of the goal), they need to feel that it is theirs—that it is about them and within their control.

- *Intentional*: The goal needs to feel motivational, to fit with the owner's values and priorities. Goal setters need to feel clear about what they will get by achieving the goal.

- *Sensorial*: The goal needs to be measurable in sensory terms. What will the individuals see, hear, and feel that lets them know they have achieved the goal?

- *Ecological*: The goal and the process of achieving the goal need to have a positive and constructive impact on the owner's self-esteem, workload, team, organisation, work-life balance, family, environment, etc. Goal setters need to understand the ripple effect (intended and potentially unintended consequences) of the goal and the action required to achieve the goal in other areas of their work-life (e.g., Ordonez et al. 2009). They need to know the priority of the goal compared to other goals. They need to know what could get in the way of the goal being achieved and what they could do to prevent the issues and/or resolve them if they happen.

- *Destined*: The goal needs to sit in the owners' timeline/time frame. They need to know when it has to be achieved by, how long it is likely to take and what that means in terms of their schedule.

Test out the POISED model for yourself. Write a goal that you would like to achieve and check it against the POISED criteria. Alternatively, refer back to your reflection earlier and write out that 'desire' as a goal. Talking with a peer to check your goal against the criteria can help to tease out even more of the detail.

# 'Objectifying' Goals: Gaining Absolute Clarity

One of the key components of a successful goal is 'clarity'. We need to be able to get specific and precise as to what we really want (in part to be able to communicate this to others). Gaining clarity is true of both the logical (SMART) and the psychological (POISED). Although SMART tells you that goals need to be 'specific', it does not necessarily tell you *how*.

A framework we use to help people get clear about goals also comes from NLP and is known as the 'meta-model' (Bandler and Grinder 1975). This framework encourages us to ask questions to get to the 'deep structure' of what people say (i.e., to delve below the words to uncover what they really mean or want).

In a nutshell, the meta-model consists of three areas of language: distortions, generalisations and deletions (refer back to Chapter 4 for more detail on the NLP communication model, where the three patterns were outlined previously). For each of these, we need to be aware of the problems they can create and ask questions to get to the specific detail we need. A simplification of the model is highlighted in Table 14.1, along with sample questions to ask.

The idea with the meta-model questions is not to be overly pedantic or fussy; it is to make sure that our goals are specific and really say what we mean them to say. Gaining clarity of both logical and psychological frameworks will give you a fuller and even more complete understanding of the goal. This will in turn make it easier to communicate the goal to others and (we believe) give you a higher chance of success. By getting clearer and closer to the real word (i.e., what we *really* want), we are 'objectifying' our goals and maximising the chance of attaining them.

Return to your goal and notice what meta-model questions arise for you to tease out even more detail.

# Motivation to Achieve Goals

## Intrinsic and Extrinsic Motivation

According to some psychologists (e.g., Ryan and Deci 2000), intrinsic motivation (coming from within) is more likely to see goals through

**Table 14.1:** Using the Meta-Model in Practice

| Meta-Model area | Description | Problematic goal language (examples) | Questions to gain clarity |
|---|---|---|---|
| Distortions | Exaggerations, interpretation and assumptions beyond the fact. Assuming cause and effect (i.e., that one thing leads to another when it might not really) can be 'fantasy' oriented and unsubstantiated, so we need to get back to reality. | (a) Raise awareness of our product by advertising. <br> (b) Make people think we are the best. <br> (c) We need to increase market share by introducing a new product. | (a) How do we know that advertising will lead to awareness? <br> (b) How will we know that people think that? <br> (c) How will a new product increase our market share? |
| Generalisations | Making 'all or nothing' statements or 'rules' that may not be useful, so we need to check for exceptions. | (a) Include everyone. <br> (b) Always sign in. <br> (c) Staff must keep tidy desks. <br> (d) Customers shouldn't have to wait. <br> (e) The competition cannot beat us. | (a) Everyone? <br> (b) Always? <br> (c) What would happen if they didn't? <br> (d) What would happen if they did? <br> (e) What would stop them from doing so? |
| Deletions | Missing information that we may need to recover. | (a) Research options. <br> (b) Improve service. <br> (c) Beat the competition. <br> (d) Produce a winning product for people to enjoy. <br> (e) Develop standards. | (a) About what? <br> (b) Compared to what? <br> (c) Which (e.g., competition)? <br> (d) How, who, what, when, where specifically? <br> (e) In what way? |

to completion. Extrinsic motivation may come from the leader in the forms of encouragement, praise and reward, but it is often the anticipation of those things *and* the self-satisfaction of doing a good job and achieving goals that makes the real difference. As the leader, you may want to ask not just 'How do I motivate this person/group?' but also 'How do I get this person/group to be self-motivated?' The second question may give you some different answers and a 'quantum leap' in performance improvement! You might also apply this to your self—how do you keep self-motivated?

## Towards and Away from Motivation

Shelle Rose Charvet (1997) suggests that 40% of people are motivated by moving *towards* positive outcomes and reward, 40% are more motivated *away* from the consequences and problems of staying as they are and the rest are somewhere in between. In NLP terms, 'towards-away from' is an example of a 'meta-program'[5] (explored previously in Chapter 2) which acts like a continuum from one extreme to the other. Some people change depending on the context, whilst others really are only motivated by seeing the positive outcomes of achieving or the negative effects of not achieving the goal. When setting the goal, it can be helpful to ask: 'What would happen if we didn't achieve this? What might we lose?' and 'What would happen if we did achieve this? What might we gain?' This would help to motivate both sides of the continuum at the start. After this however, according to Wiseman (2009), it is generally preferable to focus on what would be gained by achieving the goal, rather than dwelling on the problems of not.

### ACTIVITY

In relation to your goal:

- What will happen if you achieve your goal?
- What will happen if you don't?
- What thoughts arise and do they increase or decrease your motivation to achieve the goal?

In a working environment, people are sometimes motivated *away from* a threat of punishment or consequences, e.g., for not reaching a target—which may have budget consequences. Whilst this can provide a high level of motivation to start with, it is unlikely to result in excellence. Once the target is reached, there may be no drive to exceed the target, so we are left with mediocrity. However, by providing a positive reward (motivation *towards*) for exceeding the target we can keep motivation engaged.

### REFLECTION

What positive reward is associated with your goal—for you, for your staff, for your department and for your organisation?

## Goals Are All about States!

In the context of goal setting, what drives us to take action is *how we feel* and *how we think we will feel* by achieving the goal. One way of looking at human beings is that everything we do, we do to achieve or avoid certain states (e.g., to feel uplifted and/or avoid feeling disappointed). As a word of warning, research suggests (e.g., Street et al. 2004) that states, like happiness for example, need to remain independent of the achievement/failure of a goal: When a state is the ultimate object of a goal (e.g., 'I'll be happy only when I have done this'), it is suggested that this can be a contributing factor in the development and maintenance of depression in adults. However, states *can be* motivators on the journey to achieving the goal (i.e., be happy whilst working towards achieving the goal!).

In NLP terms, a state is not just an emotion, but also our thoughts, physiology and other mental processes at a given moment in time. The trick is to help people get into the 'right' state for working on actions to achieve the goal (see sidebar).

> ### Right State = 'End State'
>
> In order to access the 'right' state for a goal, John Overdurf (2004) has introduced the concept of 'end-state energy'. In real terms, we find the 'end state' by asking: 'How will you feel when you achieve this goal?' Whilst accessing/feeling the 'end state', ask: 'What is the next smallest step you need to take to achieve the goal?' By repeating this process as necessary, we use the motivation this provides to take us another step towards success.

## Final Word

To be effective as an individual and to create a healthy and prosperous organisation, we need to set goals logically (establish the specific outcome and how we will achieve it) *and also* set goals psychologically (gain the motivation to drive action). As leaders, through goal setting logically *and* psychologically, we can give clear direction and be flexible in being

### A Goal for Supporting Lone Worker Nurses

Although the top-level goal ('making nurses feel supported') may not have appeared to meet the SMART/POISED criteria, the means to achieve the goal were. Nurses were expected to carry the communication device and use it throughout their shift, which met the SMART criteria. The outcome was positively stated, owned by each nurse, was within their control and met their values of safety. The goal met the intention of making nurses feel supported and safe. It was sensory (measurable) in that nurses could see that they had the device with them. It was ecological in that it enhanced their safety and it was in their time frame of always carrying the device on each shift.

prepared for environmental changes. As the environment changes, our objectified, 'single point' goal may become outdated; however, the reason *why* we want to achieve the goal is less likely to change. When a goal becomes redundant, we return to the end state (i.e., why we want what we want) and reset the logical goal according to our psychological goal. From time to time we also check that our psychological goal is still valid and motivational. If it is not, we go back to the organisation's mission. If the organisation's mission is outdated, then we reset the mission. Goals can then form a valuable part of team planning and individual performance appraisal, as well as being used in your own leadership journey. This chapter gives practical advice for writing goals which are achievable and hugely increase the chance of success. It will be a chapter you return to time and time again as you refine your own methods of writing and reaching goals effectively.

## Notes

1.  This is based on nearly 20 years each of working with managers and staff on training courses and asking the question: 'What are the best and worst qualities of good and bad leaders?' The top response for poor leadership is almost consistently 'lack of direction'.
2.  For more information about Richard Wiseman's study and his findings on goal setting, see pages 88–93 of his book *59 Seconds*.
3.  Have a look online for information about SMART. A search engine check (21 February 2011) returned well over 87,000,000 hits for 'SMART goals'.
4.  For more information about NLP, see the website of the Association for Neuro-Linguistic Programming: www.anlp.org.
5.  For further information about meta-programs, see Shelle Rose Charvet's *Words That Change Minds* (1997) and *Figuring Out People* by L. Michael Hall (2005).

## References

Argyris, C. 1994. *On organisational learning*. London: Blackwell Business.

Bandler, R., and J. Grinder. 1975. *The structure of magic*. Palo Alto, CA: Science and Behavior Books.

Charvet, S. R. 1997. *Words that change minds*. Dubuque, IA: Kendall Hunt Publishing.

Day, T., and P. Tosey. 2011. Beyond SMART? A new framework for goal setting. *Curriculum Journal* 22 (4): 515–34.

Doran, G. T. 1981. There's a SMART way to write management's goals and objectives. *Management Review* 70 (11): 35–36.

Hall, L. M. 2005. *Figuring out people*. 2nd ed. Clifton, CO: Neuro-Semantic Publications.

Hartigan, I. 2012. Goal setting in stroke rehabilitation: Part 1. *British Journal of Neuroscience Nursing* 8 (2): 65–69.

Hersh, D., L. Worrall, T. Howe, S. Sherratt, and B. Davidson. 2012. SMARTER goal setting in aphasia rehabilitation. *Aphasiology* 26 (2): 220–33.

Latham, G. P., and E. A. Locke. 2006. Enhancing the benefits and overcoming the pitfalls of goal setting. *Organizational Dynamics* 35 (4): 332–40.

Locke, E. 1996. Motivation through conscious goal setting. *Applied and Preventive Psychology* 5: 117–23.

Malott, M. E. 2003. *Paradox of organizational change*. Reno, NV: Context Press.

Neck, C. P., H. Nouri, and J. L. Godwin. 2003. How self-leadership affects the goal-setting process. *Human Resource Management Review* 13 (4): 691–707.

Ordonez, L. D., M. E. Schweitzer, A. D. Galinsky, and M. H. Bazerman. 2009. Goals gone wild: The systematic side effects of over-prescribing goal setting. Harvard Business School NOM Unit Working Paper No. 09-083. http://papers.ssrn.com/sol3/papers.cfm?abstract_id=1332071.

Overdurf, J. 2004. *Beyond goals*. Audio. www.johnoverdurf.com.

Pearson, E. S. 2012. Goal setting as a health behavior change strategy in overweight and obese adults: A systematic literature review examining intervention components. *Patient Education & Counseling* 87 (1): 32–42.

Peter, L. J. 1977. *Peter's quotations: Ideas for our time*. New York: William Morrow & Co.

Ryan, R., and E. Deci. 2000. Self-determination theory and the facilitation of intrinsic motivation, social development, and well-being. *American Psychologist* 55: 68–78.

Snyder, C. R., and S. J. Lopez, eds. 2005. *Handbook of positive psychology*. Oxford: Oxford University Press.

Street, H., P. Nathan, K. Durkin, J. Morling, M. A. Dzahari, J. Carson, and E. Durkin. 2004. Understanding the relationships between well-being, goal-setting and depression in children. *Australian & New Zealand Journal of Psychiatry* 38 (3): 155–61.

Wiseman, R. 2009. *59 seconds: Think a little, change a lot*. London: Pan Macmillan.

# 15 Resilience

Gerri Power

More than education, more than experience, more than training, an individual's level of resilience will determine who succeeds and who fails. That's true in the cancer ward, it's true in the Olympics, and it's true in the boardroom.

**Dean Becker**
*President and CEO, Adaptive Learning Systems* in interview with Diane Coutu, *Harvard Business Review*

This penultimate chapter is an essential component in your leadership skills: How do you keep going when things get tough?

## The Case for Resilience

Now more than ever, resilience may be the attribute most needed in order to flourish as a healthcare professional today. Given the rapid nature of change and workplace adversity associated with funding cutbacks, increased workloads, restructuring, widespread staff shortages and the level of uncertainty in the workplace, people's stress levels are increasing exponentially. Some occupations, by definition, are more stressful than others: doctors, social workers and other caring professionals frequently suffer from high stress levels, with nurses top of the list (Wolfgang 1988). Frequently under pressure, they are challenged to respond to complex problems amidst shifting priorities as they manage the needs of a growing patient population. Health professionals constantly face change in the work they do and in how they perform the work, so it's the rare soul who doesn't feel pressured to do more with fewer resources. Add personal stress to the mix—relationship breakdowns, financial difficulties, long commutes, battling a health issue, home and family demands, job insecurity or retrenchment—and the results can take their toll, leading to disillusionment, burnout and depression. It is the life-enhancing skills of resiliency that reduce this risk, impacting positively on the daily experience of healthcare professionals.

Recognising where we sit on the continuum of stress and resilience is important to healthcare professionals who support or lead frontline staff, as a leader's attitude when confronting adversity is crucial. The ability to manage our own stress is an essential attribute, as our level of resilience amidst change directly influences the behaviour of others and their ability to be resilient to adverse events. 'Leaders are the stewards of organisational energy [resilience].... They inspire or demoralise others, first by how effectively they manage their own energy and next by how well they manage, focus, invest and renew the collective energy [resilience] of those they lead' (Loehr and Schwartz 2003). To quote Walt Whitman (1856/1900), poet, journalist and volunteer nurse during the American Civil War,

> I and mine do not convince by arguments, similes, rhymes,
> We convince by our presence. (Verse 10, lines 15–16)

Effective leadership requires resilience, the ability to provide a steady presence in charged situations or a crisis, and to demonstrate grace under pressure. Hodges et al. (2005) consider resilient nurses an essential element in an ever-changing healthcare system.

Crises tend to reveal and magnify underlying strengths as well as weaknesses. Some individuals thrive in challenging times. They focus on their strengths, enabling them to adapt to change in a healthy way that broadens their perspective and enhances their contribution. They model a capacity to engage with the difficult aspects of life rather than withdrawing when things don't go as planned, focusing their energy on the opportunities, not the constraints they face. In contrast, others, ruled by their anxieties and fears, focus on problems and get stuck in a pattern of negative thinking that narrows or limits their options. They feel overwhelmed and ineffective with a sense that they have few choices in the adverse situation (reflect again on the issue of cause and effect—Chapters 3 and 4).

Resilient leadership is a matter of continuing to grow and transform. This requires the capacity for adaptability: the skill to shift gears to respond to change or ambiguous situations, to absorb disruptive events and stay on purpose when the going gets tough. Warren Bennis (2007), widely regarded as the pioneer of the contemporary field of leadership, comments: 'I believe adaptive capacity or resilience is the single most important quality in a leader, or in anyone else for that matter, who hopes to lead a healthy, meaningful life.' (p. 5)

This chapter explores how cultivating and practising a specific group of resilient attitudes and skills strengthens the adaptive capacity, leading to new perspectives and an improved ability to manage the stressors in our life more skillfully. Based on the four cornerstones of resilience—a strong spirit, a resilient mind-set, meaning and purpose in life and understanding how our thoughts affect our emotions—the chapter offers a selection of strategies to enhance your resilience capacity. Aimed at those in formal leadership roles and those who informally lead or influence others, it emphasises the contribution resilience makes to successfully leading or navigating change and to your well-being as a healthcare professional.

This chapter shows how you can actively participate in building and strengthening a range of personal resources into your daily life to manage challenges and opportunities with greater resourcefulness and increase your well-being and life balance. Examples drawn from a composite of health professionals seen in a coaching context demonstrate how, when used effectively, these skills contribute to your ability to recover, learn from, move forward, adapt and grow when confronted with change and ongoing challenges.

# What Is Resilience?

The term *resilience* is used in a broad range of contexts including personal, community and ecological. However, there is universal agreement on the qualities that characterise a resilient individual:

- The capacity to recover, bounce back and continue forward in the face of adversity

- The ability to stay calm, mindful and focussed under pressure and uncertainty

- A high level of self-awareness

- The ability to respond flexibly and adapt to changing circumstances

- An attitude of realistic optimism and a positive perspective on life

- An ability to find meaning and purpose in life

- The ability to form strong interpersonal connections

- A mind-set that is open to learning and new experiences

We all suffer knocks to our confidence from time to time which can cause us to question the lives we've built and who we are. Think of those who have lost their jobs or a business, or who have received a serious diagnosis. Resiliency is essential to rise above adversity, as those who are resilient display a greater capacity to continue forward in the face of difficulty or a crisis. But it's much more than the ability to bounce back when our life is knocked off track, or to persevere when things go awry. Waltner-Toews et al. (2003, p. 26) have conceived resilience as a buffering process, one that may not eliminate risks or adverse conditions, but does help individuals deal with them effectively.

However, as Waller (2001) suggests, resilience is not only about crisis management, it may also reflect the concept of 'reserve capacity'. That is, a resilient mind-set helps us prepare for future adversity and enables the potential for change and continued personal growth throughout our lives. We could think of it as 'sustainable resilience', where there is a forward-leaning orientation towards engagement, purpose and perseverance throughout our lives.

## Life at the Crossroads of Change

> In the middle of the road of my life, I awoke in the dark woods where the true way was wholly lost.
>
> **Dante Alighieri,** *The Divine Comedy*

Resilience is not a new concept. History is filled with the biographies and poetry of men and women whose greatness was achieved primarily through the resilience with which they met and overcame adversity. The opening line (above) to the epic poem *The Divine Comedy*, written in the thirteenth century by the famed Italian writer Dante Aleghieri (1949), has equal relevance in the twenty-first century.[1] Dante's disconcerting words resonate with many as an apt description of the personal sense of confusion they experience when faced with disruptive change or a major life upheaval.

Although the complexity of change offers us many learning moments, it also has the potential to stir up feelings of apprehension, as people are often quite uncomfortable with change, for all sorts of reasons. With no map, and no immediate answers, the experience of change can lead to hesitancy, even resistance to enter what is perceived as the difficult terrain ahead. Uncertainty is part of life, and people differ in their responses to change and stressful circumstances. When things get tough, some people manage to carry on, whereas others are almost overwhelmed. They become troubled by anxiety and self-doubt; pessimistic thoughts of impending or past failures take their toll, resulting in a tendency to believe they don't have the resources to manage the implications of yet another change. There's a fear of getting 'lost in the dark woods'—of losing their direction, their sense of purpose, and confidence in their ability to find their way through. When these thoughts go unchecked, there is the very real danger of believing that what they do won't make a difference anyway, and they lose heart for going forward. Warren Bennis, author and founding chairman of The Leadership Institute at the University of Southern California, presents an illuminating perspective, describing the response to adversity as a leader's moment of choice:

> I suspect that we learn the most facing adversity. In my own studies, I've found that people who face adversity and grow from it have all the makings of becoming an effective leader (and person). One woman CEO I interviewed said 'It wasn't until I hit bottom twice that the iron entered my soul and turned into the steel and resilience I needed'. (Levin 2000)

Whilst not sought or welcomed, there are things we learn from hardship that we wouldn't otherwise have. The 'hitting bottom experience', as described when these leaders experienced failure or something that was personally difficult, has the potential to be transformative, to connect with the life force of resilience that transcends or rises above stressful, even traumatic circumstances.

## Can Resilience Be Learned?

Glenn Mangurian (2007), a frequent speaker to executive audiences on the subject of leadership and resilience, rebuilt his life after a spinal cord injury left him paralysed. He believes that we are born with a renewable capacity for resilience—a built-in power to heal, regenerate, and grow beyond our known limits. His article in the *Harvard Business Review* is inspiring as he describes his initial despair, his moment of truth while in hospital of finding the will to accept that his old life was gone and his determination to choose to go forward, to create an equally meaningful life in his new reality. Glenn describes how

> Some people emerge from adversity—whether a career crisis or a devastating breakup, a redundancy or a frightening diagnosis—not just changed but stronger and more content. They seem to have found new peace and even an optimism that they didn't have before. (p. 125)

Resilient people do experience monumental setbacks, as we can see from Glenn's story. It's how they respond to the adversity that makes the difference. We need to be clear that being resilient isn't about toughing it out. It doesn't mean ignoring feelings of sadness, loss or disappointment or that you will avoid any emotional scars from a trauma. Nor does it mean you always have to be strong and that you can't ask others for support. In fact, being willing to reach out to others is a key component in resilience, and Glenn's story bears witness to this. No one is immune to the arrows of life. Some will wound deeply, while others, more like darts, take the form of everyday hassles—a range of irritations, disappointments and frustrations. But when we add our reactions to these, they become 'second darts', and these are the ones we throw ourselves—at ourselves. Think of these darts as our automatic thoughts, where we run a continuous loop of negative scenarios in our mind (the inner voice discussed in Chapter 2). We pay a heavy price for this, as our moment-to-moment experience becomes one of anxiety, fear, worry and powerlessness. And this affects not only how we experience the situation in the moment, but also how we view the future. While many factors affect the development of resilience, the most important one is the attitude we adopt to deal with adversity.

So is resilience an inborn trait, or is it one that can be developed? Though there may be some genetic components to resilience, experts agree that for the most part it's a learned trait, and that no matter where you are on the continuum right now, you can strengthen your resilience. Strengthening resilience is an approach that takes time to develop, and the focus and practice of developing key attitudes and attributes has been the subject of research over the last 50 years.

# Resilience Research

How to build resilience is an exciting area of research. What is known so far suggests that the things most likely to help build resilience are cultivating positive emotions, developing an optimistic mind-set, meaning and purpose in life, and having good social support.

Resilience in the academic literature is a relatively new management focus. Its origins are rooted in developmental psychologist Emmy Werner's groundbreaking longitudinal study concerning children born into poverty and disparate life circumstances in Hawaii (Werner, Biermann and French 1971; Werner and Smith 1977) who, against all odds, not only survived adversity, but flourished. The most significant finding was that one-third of all high-risk children displayed resilience and developed into caring, competent and confident adults despite their problematic development histories. They made a successful transition to adulthood due to a cluster of protective factors that support resilience;  an active approach to problem solving, a tendency to perceive their experiences in an optimistic light, an ability to elicit positive attention from others and strong social support outside the family.

Since Warner's landmark study, numerous others have furthered the research on resilience both in children and in adults. A brief look at a few of these contributors include psychologists Salvatore Maddi and Suzanne Kobasa (1984), who in the mid-1970s through the mid-1980s helped refine the understanding of resilience with a 12-year landmark study of 450 Illinois Bell Telephone male and female managers and supervisors going through the turmoil of industry deregulation. Their findings led to the Hardiness Model, and in the following decade they co-wrote a book, *The Hardy Executive: Health under Stress*. They found that those who were resilient through this disruptive change shared three attitudes now known in the field as the three Cs of hardiness: commitment, control and challenge (Kobasa et al. 1985). They believe that what they do is important (commitment); they believe that they can influence the outcomes of events (control); and they are more likely to regard the demands of a potentially stressful event more as a challenge than as a threat. It's these beliefs that act as a buffer to protect them from the harmful effects of stress.

Studies of hardiness (Kobasa et al. 1985), self-efficacy (Bandura 1997) and optimism (Chang 1998) have all found that central to resilience are our beliefs, as our responses to stress are to a large extent determined by our thoughts and beliefs. The way we think about stress and adversity, our beliefs about our abilities and our attitudes toward the future all have powerful effects on how we cope.

Resiliency training is an outgrowth of the cognitive theories of eminent psychologists Albert Ellis and Martin Seligman and psychiatrist Aaron Beck.

Seligman, professor of psychology at the University of Pennsylvania and a past president of the American Psychological Association, is a legendary researcher in the field of learned optimism. He and his colleagues at the University of Pennsylvania studied the development of resilience for more than 30 years, identifying optimism as a key component. Most notable is their research into the habitual way in which people explain the causes of bad events to themselves. Seligman describes an explanatory style of realistic optimism, which is a powerful predictor of success and wellbeing and believes that by changing the way we think, we can change not only our outlook on life, but the quality of our life.

A body of research since 1980 has supported the theory that explanatory style predicts achievement in various domains, such as in school, work and sports. A pessimistic explanatory style has been related to lower grades in college (Peterson and Barrett 1987), lower immune system functioning (Kamen, Rodin and Seligman 1987), and it is predictive of poor health in middle and late adulthood (Peterson, Seligman and Vaillant 1988). In addition it has been very clearly linked with depression (Abramson, Seligman and Teasdale 1978).

Karen Reivich and Andrew Shatte (2002) together synthesized and built on decades of research in cognitive psychology, particularly the work of Aaron Beck and Martin Seligman, to create seven practical strategies comprised of seven abilities for enhancing our capacity to weather even the most difficult of setbacks. Their contribution through 15 years of resilience research was that the primary uses of resilience for individuals are fourfold: to overcome the obstacles and limitations of a disadvantaged childhood; to steer through the stressors and hassles in life more gracefully; to bounce back and find a way to move forward from major setbacks and life-altering events; to reach out to achieve one's highest potential and to find renewed meaning and purpose in life.

## How Resilient Are You?

When life throws us a curve ball, how is it that some people can bounce back fairly quickly while others become overwhelmed? Are there particular qualities that underpin a resilient response? Research has identified a range of important factors that constitute resilience, and Karen Reivich, PhD, and Andrew Shatte, PhD, in their work on the nature of resilience, distinguished seven key abilities that help us to manage setbacks, disappointments and major upheavals in life.

If you are to improve your leadership skills, then you should be aware of your current level of skills, your strengths and those that need development; and this book, if you have worked through the examples, will greatly help you to do that. Recognising these skills will help you to explore your relationship with resilience and will act as a benchmark as you read through this chapter. Read through the following key abilities and then score yourself on a scale from 1 to 5 (1 = low and 5 = high) by circling the relevant number.

1. Emotional awareness and control

   Entails the ability to stay calm, rein in emotions and listen when under pressure. Displays competency in a set of skills that help to regain emotional control when upset, and in choosing a resilient attitude as opposed to getting stuck in a limiting emotional pattern. Capable of expressing emotions in a healthy and constructive way.

   1    2    3    4    5

2. Impulse control

   Manages impulsive feelings and distressing emotions well, capable of deferring gratification to act in a way that will later benefit themselves and others. Ability to tolerate uncertainty, taking time to think about decisions/actions.

   1    2    3    4    5

3. Realistic optimism

   Realistic optimists combine a positive attitude with an honest assessment of the challenges that face them.  They maintain a clear-eyed view of reality while believing in their ability to solve problems and influence the direction of their life.

   1    2    3    4    5

4. Flexible thinking

   Refers to the mental ability to adjust habitual thinking in response to change and unexpected setbacks and adapt to new situations; the ability to consider many factors and view problems from a range of perspectives, others as well as your own, generate options then choose the best way forward.

   1    2    3    4    5

5. Empathy

   The ability to read and understand the behavioural cues and emotions of others, to see things through someone else's eyes. An empathetic person can temporarily shift out of his or her own perspective, and adopt the perspective of another. Empathy serves resilience by facilitating strong social relationships that provide a vital support system you can turn to when you need help.

   1    2    3    4    5

6. Self-efficacy

   Central to resilience is belief in one's self. Self-efficacy refers to the belief that one can execute given levels of performance. Resilient individuals believe that they are effective in the world and have confidence in their ability to solve problems. They know their strengths and weaknesses and rely on their strengths to navigate life's challenges.

   1    2    3    4    5

7. Reaching out

This skill involves the ability to enhance the positive aspects of life and a willingness to take on new challenges and opportunities, to try new things, to grow and expand. Failure is not seen as something to be avoided or that reaching out and asking for help is a burden to others. *They recognise they don't have to struggle and do it on their own.*

1    2    3    4    5

## REFLECTION

Self-reflection (leading to self-awareness) is key to improving your leadership potential and performance, as to effectively lead others you must first have a mature understanding of who you are and why you behave in the ways you do. Engaging in reflective journaling as you progress through this chapter and this book will promote self-awareness as you think about aspects of your experiences and your reactions to them. The reflective process aids in gaining insight into your values and behavioural patterns and in clarifying your opinions, perspectives and beliefs, and it encourages you to track patterns, trends, improvement and growth over time.

Reflect on the key resilient leadership abilities and the scores you gave yourself.

1. Make a list of your resilience strengths (scores of 4 or 5) and reflect on the way these have contributed to your personal leadership in difficult times.

2. Identify a setback or turning point you've experienced previously. What factors/strengths helped you to rise above the challenge? Describe how.

3. Consider a current workplace challenge or setback, or a significant source of stress such as a work issue or conflict, family or relationship problems, a health issue, or financial stressors. How can you use your resilience strengths more fully to cope with these?

4. Assess any areas of potential development, i.e., those resilience skills where you scored 3 or under. How would devoting some energy to these weak skills affect the way you respond to current challenges?

# The Power of Realistic Optimism

There is nothing good or bad, but thinking makes it so.

**Shakespeare,** *Hamlet* (Act 2, Scene ii)

The thinking that 'makes it so' is our explanatory style, the habitual ways we interpret what happens to us. Professor Martin Seligman (1998) found that the difference between people who give up in the face of adversity and those who persevere, is often rooted in the way they habitually explain to themselves the events that happen to them. As alluded to earlier, Seligman defines our explanatory style as one of optimism or pessimism—a way of viewing the world where you either maximize your strengths and accomplishments or you focus on your weaknesses and setbacks and make universal statements about your life when something goes badly. Everyone who has a setback or failure is stopped in their tracks, at least briefly. However, optimists recover faster, are better able to keep things in perspective and are able to act again sooner due to the way they explain the failure to themselves.

Optimism and pessimism are not characteristics that you either have or do not have; they are present in degrees. Resilience research defines optimists as positive about the future but realistic in their planning for it, with the ability to look accurately at what is happening as well as what is possible. Realistic optimists are not blind to the negative possibilities, but choose to focus on the positive, as opposed to the naiveté of a Pollyanna style of optimism—someone with unrealistic thinking, who is blindly optimistic about every situation, often to the point of foolishness. For some, their automatic reflex is to believe that a setback is long-lasting, far-reaching and their fault, and these people tend to anticipate the future as uncertain at best and, at worst, filled with continued difficulties. Excessive pessimism is an internal stressor to the body, and how we think about an event, whether it's our current reality or anticipating our future, is a huge determinant of resilience.

The three dimensions of a pessimistic explanatory style are known as the three *P*s. How we explain difficult situations to ourselves is framed across the dimensions of permanence, pervasiveness and personalization, our internal dialogue might sound like.

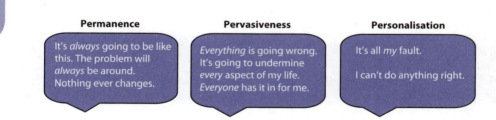

**Permanence**

It's *always* going to be like this. The problem will *always* be around. Nothing ever changes.

**Pervasiveness**

*Everything* is going wrong. It's going to undermine *every* aspect of my life. *Everyone* has it in for me.

**Personalisation**

It's all *my* fault.

I can't do anything right.

Those with a pessimistic mind-set (and internal dialogue) internalise a failure or setback. They view it as ongoing and likely to occur again (*permanent*), typical of their lives (*pervasive*), and their fault, following their tendency to excessively blame themselves when something goes wrong (*personalisation*). This 'Always, Everything, Me' explanatory style puts them at risk for depression, anxiety and low self-esteem. It is essential to step back and distance yourself from relentlessly pessimistic explanations, as this thinking directly impacts what you believe about the event and what you are capable of influencing. A pessimistic explanatory style leads to a downward spiral in confidence and a sense of helplessness; where a person becomes discouraged, believing that they cannot influence the event and that what they do will not make a difference, so they give up trying. If we explain a failure as permanent and pervasive, we project our present failure into the future and into all new situations.

In contrast, the optimists who are confronted with the same hard knocks as the pessimists weather the setbacks better. They explain a personal setback to themselves from a more encouraging viewpoint, and look for what went wrong in the situation, rather than blame themselves.

An optimistic explanatory style is based on the thinking that bad events are *temporary* setbacks, isolated to particular circumstances (*localised*). This includes looking at the wider picture to see if there are external factors that explain the event, i.e., identifying who or what else contributed to the situation (*externalising*). This isn't about finger pointing or trying to avoid your contribution to the situation, as gathering all the facts is an important criterion in problem solving. The three crucial dimensions of an optimistic mind-set are 'not always, not everything, not me'.

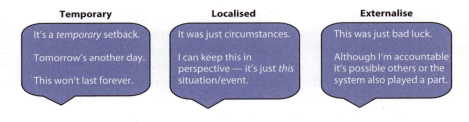

**Temporary**

It's a *temporary* setback.

Tomorrow's another day.

This won't last forever.

**Localised**

It was just circumstances.

I can keep this in perspective — it's just *this* situation/event.

**Externalise**

This was just bad luck.

Although I'm accountable it's possible others or the system also played a part.

Optimistic people expect that, in the end, things will turn out well, despite the difficulties they may face in the present, and they view themselves as less helpless in the face of stress than pessimists do. An optimistic mind-set enables them to not only learn from their mistakes and move forward, but contributes to improved health and success in the workplace and in our personal lives. Building capacity for optimistic thinking makes good sense, as it allows you to be proactive and productive in the face of setbacks or failure, to remain calm and objective and to make better decisions. Of all the personal strengths you can develop, probably none come with as many advantages as realistic optimism.

## REFLECTION

A pessimist sees the difficulty in every opportunity; an optimist sees the opportunity in every difficulty.

**Sir Winston Churchill**

To raise awareness of how your thinking is affecting your outlook on life, pay attention to how you use the 3 Ps to explain setbacks or disruptive change to yourself. Do you tend to see it as a permanent problem, one that is pervasive throughout all areas of your life, and that it is caused by your personal failings? Notice the language you use and ask yourself:

- Does how I'm explaining this reflect an optimistic or a pessimistic viewpoint?
- How does this explanatory style affect how I'm viewing the situation?
- In what way does that view affect my behaviour and the actions I take?

## ACTIVITY

Think of a current stressor in your work or personal life. What's the one step you can take to move towards becoming more mindful of the positive possibilities in this situation?

# Shifting Your Explanatory Style: The ABC Model

To shift from a pessimistic to an optimistic explanatory style, Albert Ellis, PhD, (1991) ranked as one of the most influential psychologists in history, developed the ABC approach. His model shows how to recognize our beliefs about the causes of negative events and their emotional connections. Changing our interpretation of an event, asking ourselves better questions, and disputing our automatic beliefs enable us to take more positive action. The technique helps us to change the meaning we give to an event and pushes us to analyse three aspects of the situation:

- A: stands for *adversity* (the challenge or problem you face)
- B: stands for *beliefs* (the automatic thinking running through your head about what caused the event and about the implications of the event)
- C: stands for the *consequences* of your thinking: how you feel and behave— your emotions and actions

The ABC model

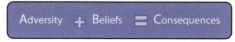

Adversity + Beliefs = Consequences

The aim of the ABC model is to help you to 'listen in' to your inner dialogue—the constant stream of thoughts running through your mind when you encounter a stressful or difficult situation. This self-talk reflects your beliefs and attitudes about the world, other people, and yourself. Identifying any thinking that can derail resilience, constrict your problem-solving abilities or tax relationships is essential to the disputing strategy. Changing the negative things we say to ourselves when we experience setbacks is a central skill of resilience. It's not what *happens* to us, but what we *say* to ourselves and how we *interpret* the event and the extent to which we believe it is possible to *influence* these events that determine our ability to absorb disruptive experiences and stay on purpose when the going gets tough.

# Disputing Strategy

Martin Seligman adapted and expanded on this technique to help us think with more realistic optimism by adding the 'D' of disputing as a strategy to challenge any inaccurate beliefs. Each time you face an adversity, listen carefully to your explanation of it. When disputing your beliefs, your aim is to move beyond your habitual way of explaining problems and approach the situation objectively, accurately and realistically.

1. *Examine the evidence objectively*: Try shifting to a 'detective role' and ask yourself what is the evidence both for and against this thinking/belief? Are these thoughts realistic? Are they in perspective? Do I have all the facts?

2. *Explore alternatives accurately*: Examine all the contributing causes and focus on those that are temporary and specific rather than permanent and pervasive. The aim is to gain a more accurate or balanced perspective in the way you view situations. Ask yourself: How can I look at this situation/ adversity from a different perspective? Am I being harder on myself than I am on other people? What might a trusted colleague say to me about this?

3. *Consider the implications realistically*: Just because a situation is unfavourable or stressful doesn't necessarily mean it's a catastrophe. Ask yourself: What is the worst/best case scenario? Examine the most realistic implications; explore what is a more likely outcome and then decide on what actions you can realistically take.

## ACTIVITY

The ABCD Model in Action

During any future adverse events you face in your daily life, listen closely for your beliefs, observe the consequences and dispute any self-limiting ones. Try this:

A. Write down the event or situation that triggered your thoughts and feelings.

B. Record the automatic thoughts that went through your head when the activating event occurred. What were you saying to yourself at the time or even after it?

C. Reflect on how you were feeling and your behaviour, how you acted. What were the consequences of the way you were thinking and explaining the event to yourself?

D. Use the steps of disputing to get a more accurate and balanced point of view.

Reflect on how the questions changed your perspective and what new opportunities opened up as a result.

## Explanatory Style and the ABCD Model
### Adversity/Situation

A senior manager in a healthcare organisation was dealing with a range of complex issues in an environment of conflict, uncertainty and increased pressure for accountability. At times exhausted and close to burnout, he expressed concern that his workload was also affecting his health, as he was exercising minimal self-care. This was taking a toll on his personal well-being and his relationships both professionally and personally. His aim in the coaching sessions was to reduce stress, increase his energy and achieve personal balance in work and life. He saw this as crucial to sustaining high performance in himself and to succeed in leading his team through change.

### Beliefs

During the coaching conversations, he became adept at recognizing that the thoughts running through his head were often inaccurate and self-sabotaging. It became evident that his explanatory style was one of pessimism, as he saw the conflict situation as never ending (*permanent*). It had started to affect his personal life (*pervasive*), and he was starting to doubt his leadership capabilities (*personalising*). His belief that 'I should be able to get through this myself' had made it difficult to reach out and admit how close to burnout he was.

### Consequences

He would often arrive late for the sessions with his mind racing. His anxiety at the possibility of failure in leading this change was palpable, and his internal conversations were harsh, critical and largely dismissive of his accomplishments, with the result that he felt trapped, frustrated and powerless. He was personalising his team's response to change and feeling responsible for events outside his control. As a result, he became more guarded and anxious in his communication, and a huge amount of energy went into comparing himself to others who, on 'face evidence', seemed to be having a 'smoother transition' through the change. This thinking fuelled a sense of inadequacy and feelings of failure.

### Strategies for Disputing a Pessimistic Explanatory Style

To renew his emotional capacity, each session began with an arrival breath meditation, which proved helpful in quieting his anxiety. It also opened him up to observations on his patterns of thinking as he began to 'hear' the most dominant themes in his conversations. The ABCD model was introduced as a means to disentangle emotions and dispute a pessimistic explanatory style. During the sessions, we explored ways to challenge his 'tunnel vision' thinking, where he tended to select and focus on the negative aspects of the situation.

*continued ...*

He increased his awareness of his explanatory style by engaging in a reflective journaling process. He began to challenge the 'always me' by asking, 'How true is that?' and looking for a more accurate explanation. Journaling also helped him in tracking his tendency to use words that exaggerate, such as *always, forever, everything*. He began to look at what were more accurate explanations, a more balanced way of seeing the situation by recalling times when he had not always been the cause of adverse events.

## Outcomes from Resilience Coaching Sessions

Harnessing the power of small wins became a confidence booster. He started to actively focus on things he did well. This increased his focus on his strengths—the times his leadership style and skills had contributed to significant and important outcomes. As a result, he became more adept at:

- Examining the evidence objectively. Reminding himself that people weren't *always* evaluating him negatively helped him keep things in perspective. Challenging the accuracy of his thinking was essential in looking for the positive side of the picture he tended to filter out.

- Staying focussed by reflecting on a series of questions including: How could I respond to this conflict or this difficulty in a way that could be more productive?

- Directing his attention to what *is* working, and noting the changes in his team when he brought an optimistic viewpoint to resolving issues and improvising solutions.

- Paying attention to his wellbeing. Strategies he found beneficial included meditation and intentional resting. (This is quite different from just lying on the couch!) It involved him rediscovering and participating in a range of healthy activities and hobbies that revitalised his energy and sense of engagement.

# Stress Hardiness

Earlier in the chapter, Maddi and Kobasa (1994) described those who not only survived but thrived through a tumultuous deregulation as sharing three qualities, now known as the three Cs of hardiness:

- *Control*: personally taking ownership of shaping our life by focusing our time and energy on what we can influence

- *Commitment*: discovering what gives meaning and purpose to our life, as it is impossible to lead an engaged life devoid of purpose

- *Challenge*: an attribute of continuous learning and growth from our experiences

These traits of hardiness help to buffer or neutralize stressful events, including those of extreme adversity. We may not be able to control what happens to us, but how we react to events is within our control. What we focus on expands as the way we think about a situation can actually diminish or enlarge the sense of personal control we have over it.

In his landmark book *Man's Search for Meaning*, Viktor Frankl (1984), an Austrian neurologist and psychiatrist, gives a compelling account of his struggles during his internment in the Auschwitz and Dachau Nazi concentration camps during World War II and, ultimately, his triumphant success in forging a life worth living. His book gives us insight into how he practised resilient leadership in such a harrowing environment. He drew on the three attributes of hardiness to not only survive the camps, but to live his purpose in life when freed and to help others realise meaning in their lives no matter their condition. In his inspirational story, Frankl recounts his struggle to hold on to hope as a prisoner in the camps, and he writes of finding a sense of purpose through, in part, imagining himself giving a lecture to an attentive audience on the psychology of the concentration camp. He believed that this method helped him rise above the despair of the moment, giving him a sense of some personal control, alleviating his sense of helplessness. He survived this grim period, bringing a remarkable perspective on the psychology of survival to his teaching and writing throughout his life (challenge). His central theme was about humanity's need for meaning, and in his book he talks about some of the inmates who carried a sense of meaning even though their life was on a perilous edge in this bleak place. Frankl believed that when we are no longer able to change a situation, we are challenged to change ourselves (control), that people can transcend or rise above stressful circumstances, and his book is a tribute to the remarkable spiritual strength and resilience many in the camps displayed.

He describes a time he was asked to speak on hope to his comrades in the camp, to offer a kind of 'medical care of their souls' while he himself was at a breaking point from exhaustion. He argues that we cannot avoid suffering, but we can choose how to cope with it, find meaning in it, and move forward with renewed purpose. Choosing to believe that life is meaningful is a commitment, particularly when events look bleak. 'In the concentration camp every circumstance conspires to make the prisoner lose his hold. All the familiar goals are snatched away. What alone remains is the ability to choose one's attitude in a given set of circumstances' (p. 12). Our circumstances are not the tragic experiences of Viktor Frankl, but his book is a testament to how we can all be leaders in our own lives, creating meaning through reaching out to others, to our community and to new opportunities even in the bleakest of times. Frankl is an example of resilient leadership, someone who said yes to life, who reached out in spite of everything.

# REFLECTION

- Have you ever experienced a leader in the healthcare sector who offered 'medical care of the soul' during tumultuous change? What did they do? What was the outcome? What insights did you gain from observing them? What can you learn from this that you can implement into your own practice?

- Reflect on a time you faced a challenging experience with your team. In what ways did you reach out to and guide them through a difficult change? What strengths and abilities did you draw on to positively influence the outcome? What did you see as your purpose at this time?

- How would practising the three components of a stress-hardy mind-set help you to:

  Manage a current or future challenge(s)?

  Thrive and flourish in your work and personal life?

**CASE STUDY**

## Stress Hardiness

### Adversity

A dedicated nurse with over 20 years' experience had lost confidence and trust in herself due to a traumatic work event. When she came to the coaching sessions, she was feeling demoralised, responsible for the event and questioning whether to continue in her nursing role.

### Beliefs/Thoughts

Using the ABC model to untangle her emotions, we explored her beliefs about the situation. We also examined her explanatory style (the 3 Ps), as dealing with negative thinking is critical as it wastes a great deal of emotional energy and is unproductive. With the ABC model, she became conscious of the thoughts that ran through her mind and listed them as:

> This work environment is too complex, it's risky. I can't concentrate or focus, what if I make another error—one that has terrible consequences? I feel responsible for what happened. I should have spoken up. How stupid of me—I'm out of my depth. I'm a failure; maybe it's time to move on. I'm sure others think that. After all these years of nursing—there goes my reputation for being vigilant in my care of patients. I'm not sure what to do; being a nurse has always been important to me.

### Consequences

This kind of thinking was damaging and exacerbating her feelings of inadequacy. Feeling overwhelmed, demoralised and lacking in confidence,

*continued ...*

her ability to sustain concentration became strained, increasing her risk for making errors. Fearful of making another mistake, she had become averse to extending herself in her professional environment and was considering less-challenging roles that felt 'safer' but did not utilize her extensive skills.

## Strategies for Disputing

The focus in the coaching sessions centred around developing the three attributes of hardiness as a buffer against stressful events; regulating negative emotions by looking for the learning and insights that arose out of this difficult experience; and considering the possibility that she was engaging in the personalising dimension of the 3 Ps, with her belief that she alone was responsible for the event. Key strategies for disputing any inaccurate thinking involved the following outcomes.

## Outcomes from Resilience Coaching Sessions

- Gained a realistic perspective on the behaviours and actions she personally needed to take ownership of in this adversity. Her explanatory style also came under focus, and she began to explore whom else, or what else, had contributed to this event, as gathering all the facts is an important criterion in problem solving and preventing a similar adverse event happening in the future. She became more mindful of each time her language reflected negative or pessimistic thinking and reminded herself how this thinking impacted on her capacity to see the range of future possibilities open to her.

- Recognition that she could shape her life positively by focusing her time and energy on what she could influence helped to shift her from a reactive to a pro-active mind-set (control).

- Recounting this adversity within the framework of the resilience models allowed her to acknowledge the learnings and insights gained from this difficult situation and, in doing this, to move forward (challenge).

- Journaling exercises were introduced that gave her valuable insight into what had drawn her to nursing and the ways this work had created meaning and purpose in her life. A particular focus was on the conversations she had with patients who were experiencing high levels of anxiety, and how the time she spent listening to their fears and reassuring them reduced this anxiety. She described these times as 'sacred moments', and there came a strong recognition that for her this was a key purpose in her nursing career (meaning and commitment).

# Mindful Resilience

I feel thin, sort of stretched, like butter scraped over too much bread.

**Bilbo Baggins, in J.R.R. Tolkien's** *The Fellowship of the Ring*

Today's workplace creates high-stress scenarios as people drive themselves to meet external demands and objectives to the extent that exhaustion becomes a huge problem. Stilling the mind is a simple and effective way to lower stress and improve memory and attention span as it calms the nervous system, increases mental clarity and lowers blood pressure. Mindfulness is a brain-training technique based on using attention to your own senses and teaches how to remain focussed in the present, alert and aware, increasing feelings of physical and mental wellbeing.

Breath awareness is a tool for managing reactions to stress. It is beneficial to the body, for when we're dealing with the breath, we're dealing not only with the air coming in and out of the lungs, but also with all the feelings of energy that course throughout the body with each breath. Feeling upset is often associated with contracted breath, so to manage your state in stressful scenarios try this simple mindfulness method.

- Sit comfortably and erect in a balanced position. Take a few moments to 'simply be'.

- Focus your awareness on your breath, staying attentive to the sensations of the inhalation and exhalation.

- Do not judge your breathing or try to change it in any way. Simply be aware of it.

- Keeping this breath awareness as an anchor, notice the thoughts that are going through your mind and any emotions. Allow these thoughts and emotions to rise and fall like waves on the ocean and notice they are continually changing, just like the breath. Don't get tangled in these thoughts, just let them float away and each time your mind wanders, gently bring it back to the breath and the body.

- In time, you will become aware of the tendencies of your mind. You will see how it resists certain thoughts and tries to hold onto others. At the end of the breath meditation, continue to be aware of your breath as you go about your various activities. In this way you can maintain a calm and clear state.

# Summary

Studies in psychology show it's not what happens to us but how we respond to an adversity that has the greatest effect on our lives. Often the cause of much of the stress and pressure that we put ourselves under comes from our own thinking—the meaning we attach to our experience. What is crucial is what we think and what we say to ourselves when we're faced with adversity or fail in an endeavour, so changing the negative things we say to ourselves when we experience setbacks is a central skill of resilience.

One of the main characteristics of resilient people is that they focus on and act upon what they have control over, choosing their attitude and giving little energy or time to factors that are beyond their sphere of influence. Resilience is not just an ability we're born with and need to survive; it is a skill that anyone can learn and improve (and a coach can help you to develop those skills over time). Taking responsibility and ownership for our own actions requires us to recognise that we are the authors of our own lives. This doesn't mean resilient people never experience setbacks or failure. They do. We only have to remember people like Viktor Frankl, Glenn Mangurian, and the great inventor and theorist Thomas Edison and many others whose names we will never know. It's what they think and do when setbacks occur that determine their resilience. Italian poet Antonio Machado (1983) expresses this attitude in a line from one of his poems.

> Last night as I lay sleeping I dreamt...that I had a beehive here inside my heart and the golden bees were making white combs and sweet honey from my old failures.

From this we can take that no experience is wasted, as our failures in life have the potential to transform us. It's as if in those moments of failure or setbacks the iron enters our soul; it is in those moments that we forge the resilience needed as leaders.

## Note

1. The author's own title for the work was simply *Comedia*. The epithet *Divina* was later applied to it by Giovanni Boccaccio, and the first printed edition to add the word *divine* to the title was that of the Venetian humanist Lodovico Dolce, published in 1555 by Gabriele Giolito de'Ferrari. It is widely considered the preeminent work of Italian literature and is seen as one of the greatest works of world literature.

## References

Abramson, L. Y., M. E. P. Seligman, and J. D. Teasdale. 1978. Learned helplessness in people: Critique and reformulation. *Journal of Abnormal Psychology* 87: 49–74.

Bandura, A.1997. *Self-Efficacy: The exercise of control*. New York: Freeman.

Beck, A. T. 1976. *Cognitive therapy and the emotional disorders*. New York: Meridian.

Becker, D. as quoted in Coutu, D. L. 2002. How resilience works. *Harvard Business Review* 80 (5): 46–55.

Bennis, W. 2007. The challenges of leadership in the modern world. *American Psychologist* 62: 2–5.

Chang, E. C. 1998. Dispositional optimism and primary and secondary appraisal of a stressor: Controlling for confounding influences and relations to coping and psychological and physical adjustment. *Journal of Personality and Social Psychology*, 74(4): 1109–1120.

Dante Alighieri. 1949. *The comedy of Dante Alighieri, the Florentine*, trans. D. Sayers and B. Reynolds. London: Penguin Books. Inferno Canto 1:160 lines 1–3.

Ellis, A. 1991. *Reason and emotion in psychotherapy*. New York: Carol.

Frankl, V. E. 1984. *Man's search for meaning*. New York: Washington Square Press/Pocket Books.

Hodges, H. F., A. C. Keeley, and E. C. Grier. 2005. Professional resilience, practise longevity, and Parse's theory for baccalaureate education. *Journal of Nursing Education* 44: 548–54.

Kamen, L. P., J. Rodin, and M. E. P. Seligman. 1987. Explanatory style and immune functioning. Unpublished manuscript. University of Pennsylvania, Philadelphia.

Kobasa, S. C., S. R. Maddi, M. C. Puccetti, and M. A. Zola. 1985. Effectiveness of hardiness, exercise and social support resources against illness. *Journal of Psychosomatic Research* 29: 525–33.

Levin, G. 2000. A conversation with Warren Bennis. *Behavior Online*. behavior.net/2000/03/a-conversation-with-warren-bennis.

Loehr, J., and T. Schwartz. 2003. *The power of full engagement*. New York: Free Press.

Machado, A. 1983. *Times alone: Selected poems of Antonio Machado*, trans. Robert Bly. Middletown, CT: Wesleyan University Press.

Maddi, S. R., and S. C. Kobasa. 1984. *The hardy executive: Health under stress*. Homewood, IL: Dow Jones-Irwin.

Mangurian, G. E. 2007. Realizing what you're made of. *Harvard Business Review*. hbr.org/2007/03/realizing-what-youre-made-of/ar/1.

Peterson, C., and I. Barrett. 1987. Explanatory style and academic performance among university freshmen. *Journal of Personality and Social Psychology* 53: 603–7.

Peterson, C., M. E. P. Seligman, and G. E. Vaillant. 1988. Pessimistic explanatory style is a risk factor for physical illness: A thirty-five year longitudinal study. *Journal of Personality and Social Psychology* 55: 23–27.

Reivich, K., and A. Shatte. 2002. *The resilience factor*. New York: Broadway Press.

Seligman, M.E.P. 1998. *Learned Optimism*. (Second ed.). New York: Pocket Books (Simon & Schuster).

Waller, M. A. 2001. Resilience in ecosystemic context: Evolution of the concept. *American Journal of Orthopsychiatry* 71 (3): 290–97.

Waltner-Toews, D., J. J. Kay, C. Neudoerffer, and T. Gittau. 2003. Perspective changes everything: Managing ecosystems from the inside out. *Frontiers in Ecology and the Environment* 1 (1): 23–30.

Werner, E. E., J. M. Bierman, and F. E. French. 1971. *The children of Kauai: A longitudinal study from the prenatal period to age 10*. Honolulu: University of Hawaii Press.

Werner, E. E. and R.S. Smith. 2001. *Journeys from childhood to midlife: Risk, resilience, and recovery*. Ithaca, NY: Cornell University Press.

Whitman, Walt. 1856/1900. *Song of the open road*. In *Leaves of grass*. http://www.poetryfoundation.org/poem/178711.

Wolfgang, A. P. 1988. Job stress in the health professions: A study of physicians, nurses and pharmacists. *Hospital Topics* 66 (4): 24–27.

# 16 Conclusions and Moving Forward

Suzanne Henwood and Grant Soosalu

At the beginning of this book, we described it as 'a personal journey of development and discovery'. With the help of some amazing authors, we have taken you through a range of components of leadership from self-awareness to resilience. We have shared case studies and prompted you to reflect and journal on how the issues we have raised impact on your own practice, the focus always being about achieving excellence in healthcare practice.

## Change Keeps Coming

Over the time it has taken to bring our thoughts together and get them into a published form, the world has already moved on. New articles and new thinking on leadership are published weekly, and the field of neuroscience and its implications for leadership are developing at a phenomenal rate. Our response to this is one of excitement, as it is evidence (as if we needed it) that the leadership journey is ongoing, with new paths and new opportunities and knowledge always opening up ahead of us. We need to stay alert to new developments, yet not be confined by new (or old) theories. We would strongly advocate a pragmatic approach to leadership which allows for flexibility and the use of what works in each individual situation and time. We see the need for both the 'art' and 'science' of leadership: moving beyond a strong knowledge base, beyond a high level of competence, to a dance in practice which enables you to weave what you know with what you feel and apply it appropriately for each person, each team and each context at any given time, always with a clear intention of optimising practice and enhancing care. No easy task, but this is what true leadership is: an organic, dynamic interplay between people, driven by a desire to make things better, fuelled by a belief that making things better is possible.

We wanted to specifically share with you the field of mBraining (mBraining.com) to show where the future of leadership coaching might be going. This is a field developed by Grant Soosalu and Marvin Oka following three years of studying neuroscience and its implications on coaching and leadership, and it is especially relevant here, as the field is largely supported and enabled through the modern imaging techniques typically used in health care. Grant and Marvin undertook extensive action research to explore the concept of humans having three brains (yes, you read that correctly). Then, over two years, they modelled experts in a variety of fields to test out their theories before launching their ideas to the literature in 2012, where they are now open to critique and further development. I will let Grant express his vision for mBraining in his own words:

### Breaking News

Over the last decade, the field of Neuroscience has uncovered that we have complex, functional and adaptive neural networks, or 'brains', in our heart and gut regions. These brains evidence memory, complex processing and their own innate intelligence, and the import of this for the field of leadership is profound! What's more, these findings give strong validation to the messages that Wisdom traditions have been telling us for over two thousand years about the importance of heart and gut intuitive intelligence, and back up what we instinctually express in the neuro-linguistics of everyday parlance through expressions such as 'learning to trust your gut wisdom', 'being true to your heart' and 'needing to digest your learnings'. And if you've ever 'lost heart', been 'gutted', had a powerful gut reaction or experienced deep intuitive messages from your heart, then you'll immediately recognise just how pervasive the intelligence and impacts of our multiple brains can be.

You see, in the increasingly complex and volatile health, social and business environments that organizations operate in, leaders who are unable to tap into and harness the full intuitive and innate intelligence of their multiple brains (head, heart and gut brains aligned together) are at a distinct disadvantage. Based on these insights and distinctions, there is a new field of leadership development that is emerging known as mBIT (multiple brain integration techniques) and it provides organisational leaders with practical methods for aligning and integrating their head, heart and gut brains for increased levels of emergent wisdom in their decision-making, and for developing an expanded core identity as an authentic leader.

Supporting this, there's also a growing body of leadership literature showing how the world's best companies are guided by leaders who can tap into the intelligence of their head, heart and guts, and who in particular are able to lead using a specific set of core competencies from the multiple brains. For example, in their popular leadership book, *Head, Heart & Guts—How the World's Best Companies Develop Complete Leaders*, leadership experts David Dotlich, Peter Cairo and Stephen Rhinesmith [2006] make the case that leaders who operate only from the head are what they consider 'incomplete leaders'. To truly thrive and lead successfully in today's complex (health), social and business environments, 'whole leaders' must learn to tap into the innate intelligence of their head, heart and guts. Backing this up, in a recent TEDx presentation, Marty Linsky [2011], co-author of several books on adaptive leadership along with Ronald Heifetz, explicitly states that 'technical leadership is from the head, and adaptive leadership is from heart and gut'.

Interestingly, all of these authors and leadership researchers have highlighted a specific set of competencies that are the domain of the head, heart and gut. These are the core skills of Compassion (heart), Creativity (head) and Courage (gut). Our work has shown that these three competencies are indeed expressed and mediated through the three brains and constitute what we call the 'Highest Expressions' of each of the brains. The Highest Expressions are synergistic and integrative and when aligned through specific techniques, generate an emergent wisdom in decision making and leadership that is truly astounding.

This is an important insight and one being supported by a growing body of evidence in the Organizational Leadership literature, along with backup from the Neuroscience of Leadership research, highlighting that the competencies of Compassion, Creativity and Courage are vital for organisational success. For example, a recent study by Christina Boedker (2012) from the Australian School of Business of more than 5600 people across 77 organisations, found that the single greatest influence on profitability and productivity was the ability of a leader to be compassionate. As Boedker observed, 'It's about valuing people and being receptive and responsive', and finding ways 'to create the right support mechanisms to allow people to be as good as they can be'. Other work in the field of behavioural economics (e.g., Gino and Ariely [2012] and Mazar, Amir and Ariely [2008]) is showing that focusing on creativity in organisations can lead to increases in cheating and anti-social behaviour. Whereas focusing on bootstrapping compassion and pro-social emotions leads to measurable increases in productivity and innovation across the organisation (e.g., Grant and Berry [2011]). All of these are important pointers to the power of the Highest Expressions of the multiple brains being facilitated and lead both within individuals at all levels of the organisation, as well as across groups and teams within the organisation.

There are also obvious and immediate applications of mBIT to organisational decision making, talent development, relationship building, coaching, and the full range of people skills that make a leader truly great. The best companies develop 'complete' leaders, and with mBIT, those leaders are able to tap into and harness the intuitive intelligence of their multiple brains to know how to wisely guide and evolve their people, their relationships, their decisions and their organisational worlds. As Dotlich, Cairo and Rhinesmith [2006] point out, great leaders turn out to be those who are deeply in touch with their head, heart and guts. Even more so, it is our view that some of the greatest gains to organisational success come from harnessing the intuitive wisdom of both leaders and those they lead, so that organisations can truly evolve and adapt with generative wisdom within our complex and rapidly changing world.

Is this the new style of leadership we have been looking for? Who could criticise a focus on wise compassion (for self, peers, employees, patients, society and the world at large)? Who would not want to evolve their workplace into somewhere where they were well respected, valued and given the opportunity to excel? Maybe mBIT is part of that solution: I certainly believe so. And that belief is the foundation of my company (mBraining4 Success) which now offers mBIT training internationally for professionals who want to find out more.

What is clear is that we live in exciting and challenging times. We are the leaders who need to ensure excellent patient care now and into the future by developing new systems and new ways of working. Numerous authors are suggesting that we need a new way of leading: We hope that this book begins to offer ways of leading differently—pragmatically, compassionately and respectfully—to meet the needs of each of us as individuals, as patients and as colleagues, as well as within the professions and organisations where we work.

## New Ways of Leading

We advocate a new way of leading which recognises and promotes the need for compassion, integrity, ethics and passionate energy to make a difference. Such a leadership honours and develops us as individual practitioners as well as recognising the service we provide. We hope that old ways of dictating to professionals, bullying and disrespectful ways of using power over others is a thing of the past, and we hope you will continue to learn and grow to ensure this. Indeed, we hope you lead this new revolution. Don't take our word for it; go and explore the literature for yourself, make your future practice evidence based. Recent research is showing what a difference such positive, pragmatic, compassionate leadership can make.

Movements such as 'Hearts in Healthcare' (heartsinhealthcare.com) established by Robyn Youngson and healthcare professionals engaging with mBraining are creating new options, new possibilities and new expectations for restoring compassion in health care. It is up to us whether we want to support, follow and contribute to and further develop these new compassionate visions to create the sort of healthcare services we can be proud of.

We should not underestimate the opportunity we have to shape the future and to inspire others who can take our plans forward to even greater heights. We hope this book has been a useful way to explore your own contribution in a new way. It is OK to get excited (and to love what you do and the thought of what you can do to be even more influential in the future). It is OK to work from a place of compassion for yourself, your patients, your colleagues, your employers and the society in which you live. It is OK to dream.

Take time out to discuss your thoughts with others, ensure that you act on your intentions and commit to making even more of a positive difference from this time on, and like I said at the beginning, let us know how things go. Go and find yourself a coach, set up a peer mentoring group, whatever it takes to ensure you keep moving forward. Put in place the support you need to make it happen and do what you can to support others along the path. We look forward to hearing your stories of how you took the ideas of this book and put them into practice: stories of your visions becoming reality and radically changing people's lives.

On a personal note, bless you for being who you are and for doing what you already do so effectively in health care. Bless you for reading this book and being open to making the quality of care even better for patients and their families. What you do and how you do it make a huge difference—we hope you take time out to recognise that and celebrate it, while continuing to strive to be the best and most compassionate you can be for your patients and for staff following behind you in their career paths. Together let's create the healthcare systems we know are possible, and ensure the best possible care for those we are here to serve.

## References

Boedker, C. 2012. *The rise of the compassionate leader*. August 21. Australian School of Business, Knowledge@AustralianSchoolOfBusiness.

Dotlich, D., P. Cairo, and S. Rhinesmith. 2006. *Head, heart and guts: How the world's best companies develop complete leaders*. New York: Wiley.

Gino, F., and D. Ariely. 2012. The dark side of creativity: Original thinkers can be more dishonest. *Journal of Personality and Social Psychology* 102 (3): 445–59.

Grant, A. M., and J. W. Berry. 2011. The necessity of others is the mother of invention: Intrinsic and prosocial motivations, perspective taking, and creativity. *Academy of Management Journal* 54 (1): 73–96.

Linsky, M. 2011. *Adaptive leadership: Leading change*. TEDx St. Charles, http://tedxtalks.ted.com/video/TEDxStCharles-Marty-Linsky-Adap.

Mazar, N., O. Amir, and D. Ariely. 2008. The dishonesty of honest people: A theory of self-concept maintenance. *Journal of Marketing Research* 45 (6): 633–44.

Soosalu, G. and M. Oka. 2012. *mBraining: Using your multiple brains to do cool stuff*. www.mbraining.com.

# Index

**Note**: Page numbers ending in "f" refer to figures. Page numbers ending in "t" refer to tables.

# Reviews

## Practical Leadership in Nursing and Health Care

### Edited by Suzanne Henwood

You could be forgiven for assuming that all of the complexities of providing modern health care come down to leadership...or a lack of it. Millions of words are written on the subject and endless varieties of training and development for health staff are available. Failings are easily attributed to poor leadership; the achievement of innovative change is seen as dependent on leadership and those who seem to demonstrate effective leadership are admired, envied and even feared. Behind all of the noise being generated is the simple truth that leadership skills are valuable tools in every-day life, transformative in any work situation and essential for anyone who calls themselves a healthcare professional.

In this book, a number of aspects of leadership in the clinical environment are examined. The approach is refreshingly practical and interactive. The assumption that leadership skills can be taught, practised and perfected is engagingly presented, with opportunities throughout for readers to reflect on their own experiences and traits in leadership. It deserves to become a resource to encourage the development of leaders at all levels in any and every healthcare service.

**Richard Evans**
*Chief Executive Officer, The Society and College of Radiographers, UK*

I have just finished reading Suzanne Henwood's book on leadership and must say that I have not been so engrossed by a leadership or management text since I studied with Russell Ackoff in the 1990s. Whereas most such books are heady and attempt to prescribe what must be done from an external perspective, Suzanne and her authors describe from the inner person how to embody the best practices in order to become a truly interactive leader and manager. The book is well designed with plentiful examples and opportunities for reflection. In every chapter there are multiple opportunities for reflection that are apt and designed to place you, the reader, into the flow of the book as participant. The examples are meaningful. It is well grounded in the history and culture of leadership and management in the healthcare professions. It is well documented and well designed for use as a textbook or a book for personal development.

**Richard M Gray**
*Research Director, NLP R and R Project, Assistant Professor (retired),*
*Fairleigh Dickinson University, USA*

A book on leadership could be a challenge to read; but not this one. The authors of this book have overcome this potential obstacle by writing in a conversational style, including questions, case studies and reflection exercises throughout.

This book will appeal to healthcare staff looking to develop their leadership skills; those wanting to bring staff together to work as an effective team and hence improve the quality of care delivered to their patients.

To be an adaptive leader, which is a must in the rapidly changing healthcare setting, we need to use the brains in our heart and gut as well as the brain in our head. The only way this will make sense to you is by reading this book; and I found that once I started reading it, I didn't want to stop. So please do read on.

**Michaela Hooper, RGN, BSc, MSc**
*Infection Prevention & Control Nurse at Frimley Park Hospital*
*NHS Foundation Trust, UK*

This timely book practises the kind of leadership that it preaches: it is refreshingly authentic, anchored in integrity and driven by a genuine desire for growth and positive change for those who work within and are served by the health sector. I congratulate the editor and the team of authors for providing such a rich multidisciplinary text that progressively integrates the freshest leadership thinking with the challenging practice of healthcare leadership.

**Professor Brad Jackson**
*Head of School of Government, Victoria University of Wellington, New Zealand*

The challenges currently facing the NHS mean leaders must widen and build on their existing strengths and expertise. Our emerging leaders need to have a range of transformational leadership behaviours and skills at their fingertips.

Improving the quality of patient care starts with leadership. It doesn't matter what you do or how experienced you are, your leadership style has the ability to inspire both staff and patients, leaving a lasting impression long after you have left an organisation.

If this book motivates just one healthcare professional to become a better leader and step up and develop their leadership and managerial skills and capacity, then it will have made a positive impact on our healthcare provision for the future.

**Caroline Shaw CBE**
*Chief Executive of The Christie NHS Foundation Trust, UK*

Many of us become health professionals because of an innate motivation to help others. Through our experiences, challenges and growing understanding in our varied roles, we strive to offer an improving service to our patients in order to equip them with relief, knowledge and the tools to be responsible for their own bodies and minds. This enlightening book allows us to grow on a personal level as well as a professional one. It does so by expanding our awareness of who we are as therapists, encouraging us to use our developing expertise to complement our colleagues and environment in order to provide the best possible treatment and outcome for each and every patient in every situation. It is also a workbook which I feel is essential to healthcare providers as a resource we can refer back to in an ongoing process of growth and continuously challenging ourselves along that journey. Each chapter is relevant and a vital part of the bigger picture with authentic and knowledgeable authors. I would recommend it on every practitioner's shelf who cares about the quality of the service they provide.

**Michelle Silvester**
*Director, Back to the Future (physiotherapy practice), New Zealand*

Leadership is an important and intriguing area—the authors have done a splendid job laying out the framework we need to address as we move forward into the future. In particular, the chapter on Coaching in Health Care brings a thoughtful and coherent group of thoughts and techniques to help those of us in the health-care field take advantage of a largely untapped resource, the 'COACH'.

**John J Sollers III, PhD**
*Psychophysiologist, University of Auckland, New Zealand*

3